ENT

Petros Koltsidopoulos
Charalampos Skoulakis
Stilianos Kountakis

ENT

Core Knowledge

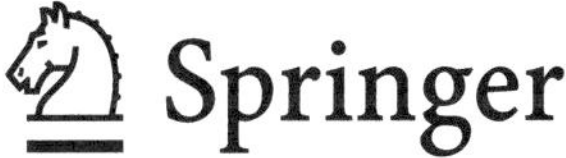 Springer

Petros Koltsidopoulos
Department of Otolaryngology-
  Head and Neck Surgery
Iaso Thessalias General Hospital
Larissa
Greece

Charalampos Skoulakis
University Hospital of Larissa
Larissa, Larissa
Greece

Stilianos Kountakis
Department of Otolaryngology-
  Head and Neck Surgery
Medical College of Georgia-
  Augusta University
Augusta, GA
USA

ISBN 978-3-319-56329-9   ISBN 978-3-319-56330-5   (eBook)
DOI 10.1007/978-3-319-56330-5

Library of Congress Control Number: 2017945401

This Springer imprint is published by Springer Nature
The registered company is Springer International Publishing AG
The registered company address is: Gewerbestrasse 11, 6330 Cham, Switzerland

Preface

Although there are many large textbooks on Otolaryngology, there is a lack of brief books suitable for revision. Thus, we decided to fill up this gap. We wrote a book that contains basic information on most of the ENT diseases; that is, we made an attempt to provide in a highly organized way the symptoms, diagnostic procedure and therapeutic approach of more than two hundred diseases.

Apart from its exceptionally brief way of structure, this book is updated with new treatment modalities, giving the reader the opportunity to keep in touch with the edge of knowledge. Moreover, we tried to make it attractive, in order to make studying easier and more pleasant, by including many images, enriching the clinical experience of the reader.

We are sure that this book would be useful for residents who are preparing for Board exams, for specialists who want to refresh and update their knowledge, and even for General Practitioners with special interest in ENT. In general, it could be an important asset for all ENT professionals as it gives them the ability to get a quick look at the basic information on most of the ENT diseases.

Larissa, Greece   Petros Koltsidopoulos
Larissa, Greece   Charalampos Skoulakis
Augusta, GA   Stilianos Kountakis

Contents

Chapter 1
Ear

1.1 Microtia-Anotia

A congenital anomaly of the ear that ranges in severity from mild structural abnormalities to complete absence of the ear, and can occur as an isolated birth defect or as part of a number of syndromes.

Classification:

- I. decreased auricle in size, normal anatomy
- II. all structures are present but there is tissue deficiency
- III. rudimentary soft tissue without recognizable structure
- IV. anotia, complete absence of pinna and canal

Syndromes associated
Treacher Collins, Goldenhar's, Pierre Robin sequence, CHARGE

Symptoms

– Conductive hearing loss up to 60 dB

P. Koltsidopoulos et al., *ENT*,
DOI 10.1007/978-3-319-56330-5_1,
© Springer International Publishing AG 2017

Therapy

1. Bone-conducting hearing aid for bilateral anotia
2. Surgical reconstruction not before 5–8 years
3. Prosthesis
4. Psychologist input if appropriate

1.2   Prominent Ears

Abnormally protruding ears.

- unilateral or bilateral

<u>Anatomic causes</u>

- underdevelopment of antihelical fold
- overdevelopment of conchal bowl
- a combination of both of these features

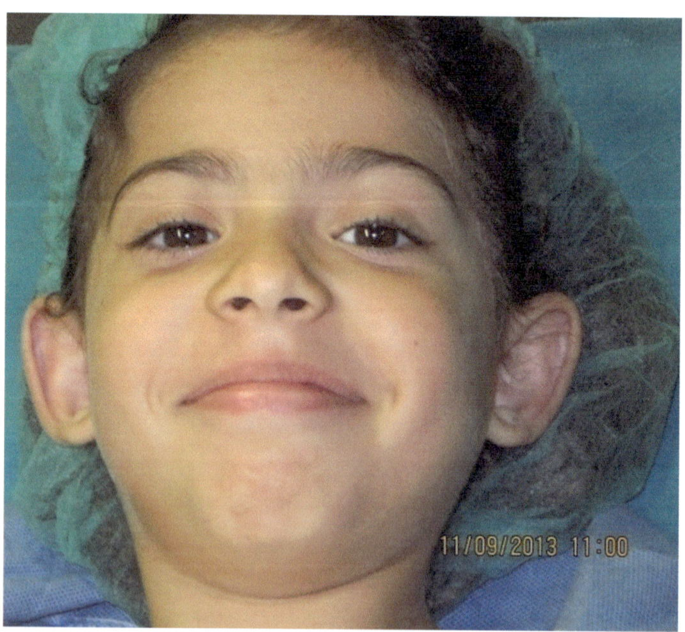

Therapy

- Ear splintage (for neonates)
- Otoplasty: suture technique by Mustarde, Incision-suture technique by Converse, Incision-scoring techniques, Cartilage thinning according to Weerda

1.3   Otitis Externa

Inflammation or infection of the skin of the external auditory canal, the auricle or both.

Pathogens: Pseudomonas aeruginosa, Staphylococcus aureus.

Predisposing factors:

1. Swimming
2. Trauma (q-tips, hearing aids)
3. Skin diseases (psoriasis, eczema)
4. Diabetes

Symptoms

- tragal tenderness
- otorrhoea
- HL
- aural fullness

Therapy

- Ear drops with antibiotics +/− steroids
- Acids: they create acidic environment and limit bacterial growth
- Gentian violet
- Pope wick (remove after 2–3 days)
- Pain management (painkillers)
- Dry ear precautions
- Regular ear cleaning
- Oral antibiotics

1.4   Otomycosis

Fungal otitis externa

<u>Pathogens</u>: Apergillus Niger (multiple black conidiophores), Candida albicans
Risk factors: prolonged topical antibiotics, diabetes, ear moisture, immunosuppression

Symptoms

Itching, otorrhoea, otalgia

Therapy

Topical antifungals, keep ears dry, regular microsuction, painkillers

1.5   Malignant External Otitis

Necrotizing infection of EAC and lateral skull base in patients with immunodeficiency

Pathogen: **Pseudomonas aeruginosa**
Risk factors: diabetes, advanced age, immunosuppression

Symptoms

- Otalgia
- Foul purulent otorrhoea
- Hearing loss

Complications

- Facial palsy (diffusion to the parotid gland)
- Palsy of IX, X, XI cranial nerves (diffusion to jugular foramen)
- Palsy of XII (diffusion to hypoglossal canal)

– Meningitis
– Epidural abscess

Diagnosis

– Otoscopy: granulation tissue in the floor of EAC
– Biopsy: to rule out malignancy
– Erythrocyte sedimentation rate: increased
– CT of temporal bones: to detect bony erosion
– Technetium-99 scan: to study the sites of osteoblastic activity (suitable for diagnosis)
– Gallium scan: to study sites of granulocytes and bacteria accumulation (used to follow treatment response)

Therapy

– Control of diabetes/correct immunodeficiency (if possible)
– Long term (6–8 weeks) treatment with quinolones
– Gallium scan every 4–6 weeks
– Analgesics/Anti-inflammatory
– Hyperbaric oxygen

1.6   Exostoses

> Broad based bony outgrowths in the osseous part of EAC

Etiology: associated with frequent cold water exposure.

Symptoms

– Hearing loss (cerumen impaction)
– Problems in drying EAC

Diagnosis

Otoscopy: multiple lesions, bilateral, broad-based, canal stenosis

Therapy

- Regular microsunction
- Surgical treatment in rare cases

1.7   Osteoma

> Benign bone mass of EAC

Diagnosis

- Otoscopy: solitary, one-sided, pedunculated mass

Therapy

- Surgical removal

1.8   External Fibrous Otitis

A form of acquired external auditory canal atresia character-ized by fibrotic tissue causing obliteration of the medial external ear canal.

Aetiology: chronic self-manipulation, chronic or recurrent external otitis, chronic myringitis, ear operations.

Symptoms

- Moderate to severe CHL
- Itching

Diagnosis

- Otoscopy:

    - EAC has a short rounded end
    - The tympanic membrane and its normal landmarks are not visible
- CT: to evaluate the thickness of the stenotic part

Therapy

– Early cases: removal of granulations and steroid cream
– Stabilized cases: surgery with high risk of recurrence.

1.9   Keratosis Obturans

Accumulation of desquamated keratin in the bony portion of EAC.

Pathogenesis: altered mechanism of epithelial migration.

Symptoms

– Conductive Hearing Loss (CHL)
– Acute ear pain
– It may cause circumferential bony widening.

Diagnosis

• Otoscopy: A large plug of keratin occludes the EAC, widening of bony EAC

Therapy

– The plug should be removed in the office or in the operating room
– Regular microsuction

1.10   Traumatic Perforation of Tympanic Membrane

Pathogenesis

• Direct trauma: cotton bud, matchsticks
• Indirect: explosion(overpressure), barotrauma, violent blow to the ear, temporal bone fracture

Symptoms

- Conductive hearing loss
- Sudden pain
- Tinnitus
- Blood discharge

Diagnosis

- Otoscopy
- Audiogram: conductive hearing loss

Therapy
<u>Conservative</u>

- Regular observation: high rates of spontaneous recovery

<u>Surgical</u>

A. Small

- Tympanic membrane patch
- Fat tissue application myringoplasty

B. Large

- Myringoplasty

1.11   Myringitis

Infection of the lateral surface of the TM.

<u>Types</u>

1. Viral (influenza virus): red vesicles
2. Granular (local trauma): pyogenic granulations
3. External (during external otitis): symptoms of external otitia
4. Tympanogenic (during AOM): symptoms of AOM

Symptoms

Otalgia, otorrhoea, aural fullness

Diagnosis

Ear microscopy

Therapy

– Puncture of vesicles
– Analgesics
– Removal of granulations and stop manipulation
– Treatment of external otitis or AOM

1.12   Otitis Media with Effusion

Accumulation of non-purulent fluid within the middle ear caused by malfunction of the Eustachean tube.

Aetiology:

– Recurrent URIs
– Adenoid hypertrophy
– Nasopharyngeal tumor
– Cleft palate
– Allergy
– Chronic rhinosinusitis
– Environmental smoking
– Nasal packing
– Radiotherapy

Symptoms

– Conductive Hearing Loss (CHL)
– Ear fullness
– Short episodes of earache
– Tinnitus

Complications

– Recurrent AOM
– Retraction pockets
– Cholesteatoma

Diagnosis

- Ear microscopy:
  - Retracted TM, fluid disc, air bubbles
- Tympanometry: type b
- Audiometry: conductive hearing loss
- Endoscopy of nasopharynx: to rule out nasopharyngeal pathology.

Therapy
Conservative

- Antibiotics
- Decongestants
- Antihistamines
- Eustachean tube exercises

Surgical

- Myringotomy
- Insertion of ventilation tubes: Bilateral OME >3 months, unilateral OME >6 months
- Adenoidectomy

1.13   Acute Otitis Media

A bacterial or viral inflammation of the middle ear cavity.

- Children prone to AOM: Shorter, narrower, more horizontal eustachian tube

<u>Pathogens</u>: **Streptococcus pneumoniae, Haemophilus influenza, Moraxella catarrhalis**

<u>Risk factors</u>: Gender, bottle feeding, sibling history of OM, daycare attendance, lower socioeconomic status, maternal smoking, craniofacial abnormalities, immunodeficiency

Symptoms

– Otalgia
– Ear discharge
– Hearing loss

Complications

– Adhesive otitis media
– Retraction of tympanic membrane
– Chronic suppurative otitis media
– Tympanic membrane perforation
– Tympanosclerosis
– Cholesteatoma
– Mastoiditis

Diagnosis

– Otoscopy

Therapy

– Antibiotic therapy
– Adenoidectomy: in case of eustachian tube dysfunction
– Myringotomy ± tympanostomy tube placement: AOM in a seriously ill or toxic child, AOM unresponsive to antibiotics, complications of AOM, AOM in an immunocompromised patient or in a newborn
– Indications for tympanostomy tube placement:
  Recurrent AOM (>3 episodes in 6 months, >4 episodes in 12 months)
  Bilateral OME >3 months, unilateral OME >6 months

1.14   Complications of Acute Otitis Media

1. **Labyrinthine fistula**: abnormal opening in the bony capsule of the inner ear
   – Fistula test: Dizziness produced by pressure on the tragus (Hennebert's sign).
   – Risk of sensorineural hearing loss with removal of cholesteatoma sac

2. **Serous inflammatory labyrinthitis.**
   - Vestibular symptoms: vertigo, nausea, vomiting, spontaneous nystagmus towards the infected ear (irritative) becomes nystagmus towards the opposite ear (paralytic).
   - Cochlear symptoms: SNHL greater for high-frequency tones, diplacusis.

Therapy
   - Caused by an AOM: antibiotic therapy and myringotomy.
   - Caused by a cholesteatoma: mastoidectomy and antibiotic treatment.

3. **Suppurative inflammatory labyrinthitis**:
   - Similar symptoms with those of serous labyrinthitis but with a more abrupt onset.
   - It can lead to labyrinthitis ossificans

Therapy

   - Antibiotic treatment and close observation
   - In case of appearance of any meningeal sign: CSF examination followed by surgical drainage of labyrinth.
   - Suppurative labyrinthitis secondary to meningitis doesn't require drainage of labyrinth.

4. **Petrositis**: suppurative bacterial infection causing destruction of bony septae of petrous apex air cells

   - Pain
     (a) anterior petrositis: frontal or retro-orbital pain.
     (b) Posterior petrositis: occipital, parietal or temporal pain.
        - Persistent otorrhoea following a simple mastoidectomy.
        - Diplopia due to abducen's nerve paralysis (CN VI travels adjacent to petrous apex in Dorello's canal)
     - Otorrhea, headache and abducen's nerve weakness constitute Gradenigo's syndrome.

- Imaging: CT air cell coalescence; T1 intermediate signal, does not enhance; T2 high signal

Therapy

- Intravenous antibiotics, ventilation tube, mastoidectomy.

5. **Facial paralysis**: complication of AOM (through a dehiscence of the Fallopian canal) or chronic otitis media (onset of symptoms often slow and progressive).

   - Incidence with acute otitis media is 0.05%

Therapy

A. Paralysis caused by AOM: myringotomy, ventilation tube insertion followed by antibiotic drops.
B. Paralysis caused by chronic OM: surgical decompression with mastoidectomy.

6. **Subperiosteal abscess**: a relatively uncommon complication in the antibiotic era. It is usually associated with the development of acute mastoiditis following an episode of AOM. Characterized by destruction of cortical bone overlying mastoid with auricle protrusion and loss of postauricular sulcus.

Therapy

- Drainage of the abscess (myringotomy and placement of ventilation tube)
- Cortical mastoidectomy

7. **Meningitis**: pyogenic infection of the pia arachnoid over the entire brain and spinal cord with viable organisms in CSF.

   Pathogens: Streptococcus pneumoniae, Neisseria meningitis, H. influenzae type B a risk in infants but vaccine has reduced incidence
   Risk factors: congenital inner ear malformations, cochlear implant recipients
   - It results from chronic otitis media in adults, and from AOM in children.

- Symptoms: headache, high temperature, photophobia, stiff neck, convulsions (esp. in children), irritability, drowsiness, ocular paralyses.
- Signs.

Neck rigidity (chin does not touch the chest).
Kernig's sign (inability to extend the leg completely with the thigh flexed on the abdomen).
Brudzinski's sign (flexion of the hip and knee when the neck is bent).
Babinski's sign (extension of the toes instead of flexion on stimulating the sole of the foot).

- Lumbar puncture: high pressure, opaque CSF, containing ≥ 1000 cells/mm^3 (polymorphonuclear), increased protein concentration, reduced glucose level, organisms in cultures.
- CT to ensure no impending brain herniation from increased intracranial pressure present

Therapy
Appropriate antibiotic treatment
Dexamethasone
Lumbar or ventricular punctures.
Surgical intervention if not responding to antibiotics alone (myringotomy with placement of ventilation tube, tympanomastoidectomy)
Complications
Sensorineural hearing loss (10–20% of infants)
Labyrinthitis ossificans: ossification prevents the ability to place cochlear implant.

8. **Lateral sinus thrombosis**:

- Spread of inflammation from the middle ear to the sigmoid sinus causing thrombophlebitis
    - Pathogens: haemolytic streptococcus, type III pneumococcus or staphylococcus.
    - Symptoms: spiking fevers ("picket-fence" temperature chart), headache.
    - CT: bony erosion over sigmoid
    - MRI/MRV: filling defect/no flow through sinus

- Progressive anaemia, especially rapid and pronounced in haemolytic streptococcal infection.
- Eye-ground changes (papilloedema).
- Oedema over the posterior aspect of the mastoid process due to thrombosis of the mastoid emissary vein (Griesinger's sign: less common symptom).

Therapy
- Intravenous antibiotics.
- A complete simple mastoidectomy or a radical mastoidectomy if the patient had chronic otitis media with cholesteatoma.
- Mastoidectomy with removal of infected thrombosis
- Use of anticoagulant therapy is controversial.

9. **Otitic hydrocephalus**: increased intracranial pressure from impaired venous sinus thrombosis.

   Symptoms: chronic headache (the most constant symptom), abducens palsy, lethargy, and vomiting.
   Signs: Papilloedema, CSF pressure exceeding 300 mL water [CSF is clear, without increase in cells or protein (unlike localized meningitis)], No localized neurological signs, (in contrast to brain abscess), CT shows no space-occupying lesions, MRI.

   Therapy
   Steroids
   Acetazolamide
   Repeated lumbar or ventricular punctures or placement of a lumbar drain.

10. **Extradural abscess**: collection of pus and granulation tissue between the dura mater and cranial bone.
    - It has an insidious onset, with symptoms developing over several weeks to months.
    - Persistent headache (ipsilateral).
    - Profuse or intermittent pulsating otorrhoea accentuated by compression of the internal jugular vein.
    - Low-grade fever of unknown origin following AOM.
    - Signs of meningismus (Kernig's, Brudzinski's).

- Recurrent attacks of generalized non-meningococcic meningitis.
- Lumbar puncture (CSF): increased white cell count, but usually with lymphocyte predominance. Glucose level normal, no organisms.
- MRI: epidural collection with strong peripheral contrast enhancement.
- **Therapy**
- Simple or radical mastoidectomy with cautious exploration of a necrotic lead to a subdural abscess or a brain abscess.
- Antibiotic therapy to prevent postoperative spreading of infection.

11. **Brain abscess.**

- Initially non-specific symptoms
  - Persistent headache refractory to analgesics
  - Nausea and vomiting.
  - Drowsiness or irritability
  - Seizures (in 30–50% of patients).

- Signs
  - Low-grade or high-grade fever
  - Intermittent slowing of the pulse, due to pressure on the vagus centre in the brainstem.
  - Eye-ground signs of increased intracranial pressure occur in about half of the cases, with blurring of the disc margins, hyperanemia or papilloedema
  - Cheyne–Stokes respiration, elevation of the blood pressure
- Localized neurologic signs are eventually found in most patients.
  - Aphasia (left temporal lobe abscess in a right-handed patient), paresis of face and mouth on the opposite side (central type, not affecting the frontal muscle), visual field defects.

Diagnosis

CT with contrast: a brain abscess appears as a hypodense area surrounded by an enhanced ring (the so-called ring sign).

MRI: There is better contrast between the area of the peripheral oedema and the surrounding brain.

CSF is rarely normal, with a slight increase in cells and protein.

Therapy

Intravenous antibiotics

Neurosurgical drainage

Ear is approached surgically at the same time or 3–4 days after craniotomy.

Dexamethazone intravenously.

Mannitol.

1.15   Acute Mastoiditis

A complication of otitis media in which infection in the middle ear cavity involves the mucoperiosteum and bony septa of the mastoid air cells.

– The most common complication of acute otitis media

Causative bacteria:

1. Streptococcus pneumonia (30%),
2. Haemophilus influenza (20%),
3. Staphylococcus aureus (20%)

- Acute mastoiditis: a few days to 1–2 weeks after the onset of untreated AOM. A postauricular subperiosteal abscess may develop (subperiosteal abscess)
- Masked mastoiditis: Chronic inflammation of mucous membrane without abscess formation.

Symptoms

- Otalgia with pain over the mastoid
- Fever
- Hearing Loss (HL)

  – These symptoms can be masked by insufficient previous antibiotic therapy (masked mastoiditis)

Complications

- Facial palsy
- Meningitis
- Labyrinthitis
- Petrositis (osteomyelitis of the temporal bone)
- Thrombosis of the sigmoid sinus
- Bezold descending abscess (spreading of the abscess into the neck muscles)

Diagnosis

- Inspection:

    - Postauricular erythema, tenderness, swelling.
    - The pinna is pushed forwards and inferiorly.

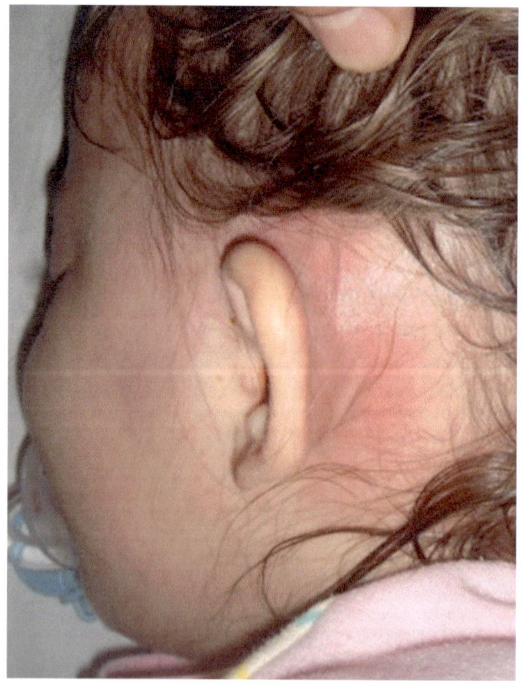

- Otoscopy:
  - Red, bulging TM or opacity due to a middle ear effusion.
  - Central perforation of the TM with purulent secretion.
  - Sagging of the postero-superior meatal wall.
- Audiogram: HL
- X-ray: Schueller projection (reduced pneumatization, cloudiness of mastoid air cell system and formation of abscess cavities).
- CT scan: opaque mastoid air cells due to purulent fluid, swollen mucosa and granulation tissue.

Therapy

Conservative

  - Antibiotic therapy for at least 2 weeks.
  - Antibiotics stable to β-lactamase, with penetration into the CNS (if a complication seems impending) +culture

Surgical

- Myringotomy with or without insertion of grommets.
- Cortical mastoidectomy (if there is no improvement after antibiotic therapy or in the case of subperiostal abscess).

1.16   Chronic Otitis Media

Chronic inflammation of middle ear mucosa characterized by a long-standing central perforation of TM with permanent or intermittent drainage (active and inactive stages).

Risk factors: recurrent middle ear infections, recurrent adenoid infections, chronic rhinosinusitis, adenoid hypertrophy, impaired nasal respiration (septal deviation, allergy), cleft palate, collagen diseases and ciliary paresis of tubal mucosa (Kartagener syndrome), severe traumatic perforations, acute necrotizing otitis media (rare) and immune deficiency.

<u>Pathogens</u>: (1) Pseudomonas aeruginosa (60–80%), (2) Staphylococcus aureus (10–25%), (3) Proteus (10–20%).

Symptoms

Recurrent episodes of otorrhoea.
In the active stages: mucopurulent and odourless secretion.

These episodes of reactivation are initiated by URIs, or by external auditory canal manipulations, or by penetration of water in the ear.

– In inactive stages: only CHL and a dry central perforation.

Complications

- Ossicular resorption (most frequently the long process of incus)
- Ossicular fixation (most frequently malleus head).

- Tympanosclerosis: hyalinized collagen changes of the middle ear mucosa limited to the TM, less frequently, extended to the ossicles (fixation and CHL) and to the promontorium.
- [Small tympanosclerotic plaques confined to the TM do not affect hearing, but a severe CHL and even a severe mixed HL may be present in extensive forms (with promontorial and stapes involvement)].
- CHL or mixed HL (inner ear toxic involvement).
- External otitis and eczema.

Diagnosis

Otoscopy: location and size of perforation, calcifications, presence of the annulus, integrity of the ossicular chain.
In inactive stages the middle ear may be perfectly dry with the margins of the perforation covered with a healed epithelium.
In active stages the central perforation is surrounded by a ring of granulation tissue and a yellowish mucopurulent exudate can be seen draining in the EAC

Hearing examination (tuning fork tests and audiometry): CHL; SNHL is not common but possible.

X-ray (Schuller) examination to assess the degree of mastoid pneumatization

High-resolution CT (hidden cholesteatoma?)

Nasopharyngeal fibroscopy

Therapy

Conservative Therapy

- Periodic cleaning of ear by local suction.
- Topical antibiotic therapy: quinolone eardrops applied for 10 days (avoid drops with ototoxic potential).
- Oral or intravenous antibiotics

Surgery

1. Dry perforation: tympanoplasty without mastoidectomy:
   - Endaural approach: large external auditory canal, posterior perforation
   - Retroauricular approach: narroe EAC, anterior perforation masked by a prominent anterior wall.
2. Persistent discharge: tympanoplasty with mastoidectomy: if suppurative drainage persists and the mucosa of the mastoid is involved.

1.17   Cholesteatoma

Presence of keratinizing stratified squamous epithelium within the middle ear cleft.

- It consists of a *matrix* which continually desquamates and of sheets of exfoliated *keratin debris* which accumulate and form the bulk of cholesteatoma.

Types

Congenital: originating from embryonic epithelial rests of ectodermal origin in the petrous bone.

Primary acquired: prolonged Eustachean tube dysfunction → chronic negative pressure in the middle ear cavity → retraction of Tμ in posterosuperior part → Local inflammation processes (*Pseudomonas aeruginosa* and *Bacillus proteus*) stimulate the growth of the cholesteatoma.

Secondary acquired: Keratinized epithelium of the EAC migrates inside the middle ear cavity from margin of an "unsafe" *perforation (destruction of the fibrous annulus).*

[Post-traumatic, Cholesteatoma from ventilating tubes]

Symptoms

- Often asymptomatic for years: the accumulation of keratin in dry cholesteatoma is slow. However, infected cholesteatomas may grow quickly.
- *Otorrhoea*: foul discharge.
- *Earache*: caused by inflammation of the meatal.
- *Hearing loss*
- *Tinnitus*
- *Dizziness*: in case of labyrinthine fistula
- *Headache*: in case of intra-cranial extension.

Complications

- *Ossicular chain lesions*
- *Labyrinthine fistula*
- *Acute labyrinthitis*
- *Facial palsy*
- *Sensorineural HL*
- *Intracranial complications*: meningitis, epidural, subdural or brain abscess, lateral sinus thrombosis.

Diagnosis

- *Otoscopy*: cholesteatoma may be visualized through attic or marginal perforation. Congenital: a white cyst behind an intact TM.

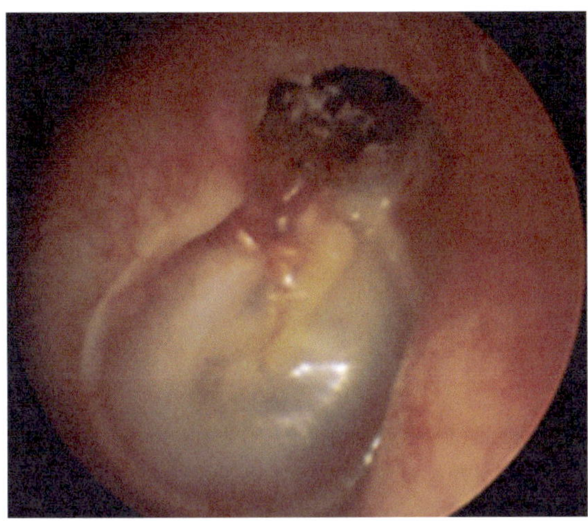

- *Audiometry*: CHL (or SNHL)
- *High-resolution CT scan*
  - defines the location of the lesion and evaluates the size.
  - provides information on the integrity of the ossicles, lateral semicircular canal, cochlea, tegmen.
  - <u>blunting of the scutum</u> (the upper bony edge of the external auditory canal).

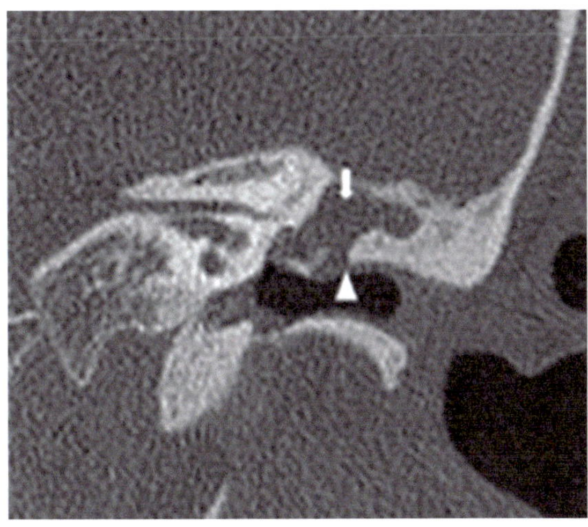

- *MRI*: if there is suspicion of intrapetrous extension or intracranial complications
- *Fistula test*: in case of suspicion of labyrinthine fistula.

Therapy
Conservative

Periodic observation: in limited cases of a dry cholesteatoma

1. only hearing ear
2. in elderly patients
3. in individuals in poor health.

Surgical

Primary goal: eradication of the disease.

Secondary goal: reconstruction of the ossicular chain immediately or at a later stage.

- *Close technique* (*canal wall up*): in children with a well-pneumatized mastoid.
- *Open technique* (*canal wall down*): indicated in sclerotic mastoids and in revision surgery for recurrences.

1.18   Barotrauma

Injury of middle ear mucosa caused by rapid or extreme changes in air pressure.

- During aircraft flights
- During scuba diving

Symptoms

- Earache
- Ear fullness
- Hearing loss
- Tinnitus
- Vertigo

Complications

– Perilymphatic fistula

Diagnosis

- Otoscopy: retracted TM, clear or haemorrhagic fluid
- Tympanometry: negative pressure
- Audiogram
- Frenzel glasses
- Fistula test

Therapy

– Nasal decongestants
– Valsava manoeuvre
– Persistent: myringotomy with insertion of grommet

1.19   Patulous Eustachean Tube (PET)

Eustachean tube remains permanently open, causing an abnormal flow of air from the nasopharynx to the middle ear during breathing.

Conditions associated with PET: Pregnancy, hormone therapy, significant weight loss, radiation therapy, fatigue, stress.
→Eustachean tube also serves to dampen the intensity at which we hear our own voice.

Symptoms

- Autophony (the most common symptom)
- Breath synchronous tinnitus
- Pressure sensation in the ear
- Hearing loss.

    – Worsening of symptoms

- Whilst standing, use of topical or systemic decongestants, exercise and anxiety.

    – Improvement of symptoms

- In situations which increase venous congestion in the peri-tubular area, such as the supine position, flexion of the thorax over the legs while seated or nasal and postnasal mucosal congestion.

Diagnosis

- Otoscopy: mobility of the tympanic membrane that occurs with respiration.

Therapy
Conservative Therapy

- Regain weight
- Oestrogen (premarin) nasal drops

Surgical Treatment

- Pressure equalization tube: may worsen symptoms
- Plugging of eustachian tube with fat or cartilage
- Paraffin or gelfoam or calcium hydroxylapatite injection at Eustachian tube orifice
- Eustachian tube occlusion with catheter (reversible, can be removed at any time)

1.20   Otosclerosis

Metabolic bone disease of certain regions of otic capsule that causes stapes fixation.

- Sites of predilection:
    - Anterior to the oval window (fissula ante fenestrum): the commonest site affected.
    - Round window
    - Promontory
    - Cochlea
- Autosomal dominant with incomplete penetrance.
- Aetiology: it is associated with local measles virus and with pregnancy.

Symptoms

– Progressive hearing loss
– Paracusis willis: improved hearing in background noise
– Tinnitus
– SNHL and vestibular symptoms: reflect involvement of cochlea

Diagnosis

- Otoscopy: normal tympanic membrane, thickened and hyperhaemic middle ear mucosa in the region of promontory (Schwartze sign)
- Audiometry: CHL or mixed HL, Carhart's notch (elevation of BC threshold at 2 kHZ, reverses after stapedectomy)
- Speech audiogram: poor speech discrimination indicates cochlear otosclerosis.
- Tymp: type As
- Absent stapedial reflex
- Gelle test: negative
- HR CT: visualization of otospongiotic foci

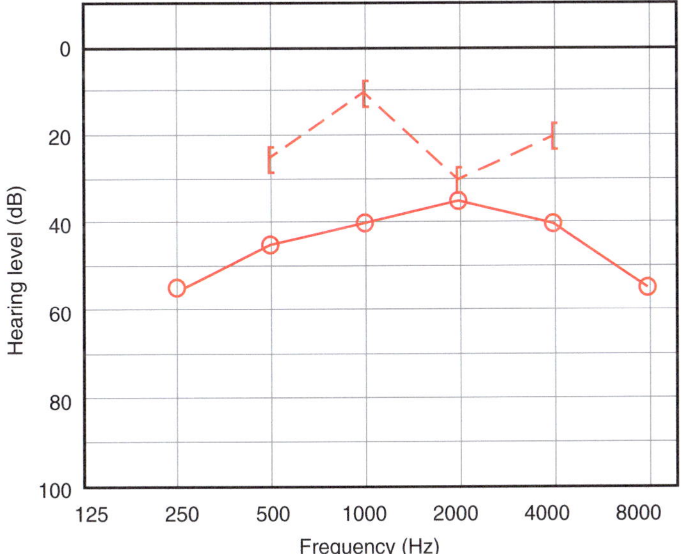

Differential Diagnosis

- Postinflammatory necrosis of long process of incus.
- Aseptic necrosis of long process of incus.
- Post-traumatic interruption or fixation of ossicular chain.
- Malleus head fixation, calcification of the anterior malleus ligament.
- Congenital ossicular anomalies.
- Superior semicircular canal dehiscence.
- der Hoeve syndrome (osteogenesis imperfect): stapes footplate fixation, blue sclerae, pathologic bone fractures.
- Paget's disease.

Therapy
Conservative

- No treatment (CHL <20 dB)
- Hearing aid (last hearing ear)

Surgical

- Stapedotomy or stapedectomy (replacing the stapes with prosthesis).

Surgical Complications

- Prosthesis displacement (most common)
- Necrosis of long process of incus
- Dead ear (1%)
- Facial nerve paralysis
- Perilymph gusher
- Reparative granuloma (initial improvement followed by deterioration)
- Permanent vertigo (too long prosthesis)

1.21   Traumatisms of Temporal Bone

Blunt, open or ballistic trauma of the temporal bone resulting in a simple concussion or a fracture of the temporal bone.

Symptoms

- Otalgia
- Bloody discharge
- Hearing loss
- Wound or a haematoma near the auricle.

Complications

- Facial nerve palsy: immediate (due to the trauma itself) or delayed (due to neural oedema or to HVS reactivation in the geniculate ganglion).
- Abducens nerve palsy (less than 1%)
- Ossicular fracture or dislocation (persistent conductive or mixed hearing loss after resorption of haemotympanum). Incudostapedial joint disjunction is the most common lesion.
- Perilymphatic fistula.
- Labyrinthine concussion: moderate to severe SNHL, unsteadiness and tinnitus without any fracture line near the inner ear.
- SNHL: it is common, going from a high-frequency HL to a dead ear—it is observed in transverse trans-labyrinthine fractures.
- CSF fistula: abundant clear or pink ear discharge.
- Meningitis (months or years after the fracture—late complication).
- Vascular compromises (carotid cavernous fistula, sigmoid sinus thrombosis, internal carotid artery rupture).

Diagnosis

- Inspection: ear canal discharge (blood, CSF), haematomas, wound, bullet penetration.
- Battle's sign: ecchymosis around the mastoid process. This sign can suggest that a patient has sustained a significant blow to the skull, even if the medical history is obscure.
- Otoscopy: blood discharge and clots in the external auditory canal, check the tympanic bone (bone fragments, stenosis) and check the TM (perforation, haemotympanum).
- Hearing examination: Hearing disorders are observed in 70% of cases.

- Frenzel glasses: to look for nystagmus and exclude vestibular irritation or loss.
- Examination of cranial nerves with a specific attention to the facial. Abducens and last cranial nerves are also checked.
- Eye examination: look for dry eye, pulsatile exophtalmos (carotid cavernous fistula), and Horner's syndrome.
- Complete neurological examination and evaluation of the level of consciousness (Glasgow score) is mandatory, as is looking for meningitis symptoms (fever, headache, vomiting and nausea, neck tenderness).
- Examination of temporo-mandibular joint function.
- HR-CT scan: The fracture line is usually classified as oblique (75%), transverse (13%) or longitudinal (12%), with regard to the great axis of the petrous bone. It can also be described as labyrinthine (more often than not transverse, crossing the otic capsule) or extralabyrinthine.
- More complex fractures (comminute) can be observed.

Therapy
Conservative treatment

- Close clinical survey for at least 3 days (secondary onset of facial paralysis, deafness, vertigo)
- Painkillers
- Microsunction of the meautus
- Calibration of the ear canal using Pope-wicks in case of stenosis.
- Collection of ear discharge: in case of suspicion of CSF leak
- Antibiotics

Surgical treatment

- Exploration of an EAC stenosis to remove bone fragments occluding the lumen.
- Emergency exploratory tympanotomy in case of suspicion of perilymphatic fistula (vertigo, dizziness, sloping HL, air bubble in the labyrinth at CT scan or MRI)
- Surgical treatment of CSF fistulas is rarely necessary [95% of cases heal within 1 week spontaneously (in case of trauma to the roof)]. Translabyrinthine fractures can cross

the IAC and lead to a productive leakage that must be sealed using a middle ear exclusion technique.
- Closure of TM perforation
- Treatment of facial paralysis

1.22 Squamous Cell Carcinoma of the Temporal Bone

– Arises from skin of EAC or from middle ear cleft
– The most common type of primary cancer in the EAC.
– Other types of carcinoma: Adenocarcinoma, melanoma, rhabdomyosarcoma, osteosarcoma, lymphoma, adenoid cystic carcinoma, and acinic cell carcinoma

Symptoms

– Otalgia
– Otorrhea
– Hearing loss
– Facial paralysis
– Bleeding
– External auditory canal mass

Diagnosis

- Otoscopy: ulcerated papillomatous lesion
- Biopsy of the lesion
- Palpation of PG and cervical nodes areas
- CT scan/MRI: localize the tumor, check for intra or extra-cranial extension.

Therapy
Conservative

– Radiotherapy (palliative): extended and aggressive tumours.

Surgical

– Lateral temporal bone resection (T1, T2)
– Extended temporal bone resection with parotidectomy and supra-omohyoid ND (T2–T4)

1.23   Vestibular Schwannoma

A benign, usually slow-growing tumor that develops from the Schwann cells of vestibular nerve within the IAC.

- Account for 80% of CPA tumors
- Grows slowly (0–3 mm per year)
- Either sporadic (95%) or part of Neuro-fibromatosis type 2 (5%)

Symptoms

- Unilateral progressive hearing loss
- Unilateral sudden SNHL
- Unilateral tinnitus
- Mild balance disturbance

Diagnosis

- PT audiometry: unilateral high frequency SNHL
- SD test: discrimination worse than expected from audiogram
- Auditory brainstem response: the most sensitive audiological test
- MRI: in contrast-enhanced T1 weighed images
- CT with contrast: visualization of medium or large VSs sensitivity of posterior wall of the ear canal.

Therapy
Conservative

- Watchful waiting: in older patients and in patients with poor health.
- Annual imaging
- Stereotactic radiosurgery (gamma knife) in small bilateral lesions (may stop the growth)

Surgical

- Translabyrinthine approach: medium size and large lesions, small lesion with poor hearing
- Middle fossa approach: small tumors with good hearing
- Retrolabyrinthine or retrosigmoidalappr: large extracanalicular lesions

Surgical Complications: deafness, facial palsy, dizziness, CSF leak, meningitis

1.24   Meningioma

Benign tumor arising from arachnoid cells

- The second most common tumors of the cerebellopontine angle (CPA) after vestibular schwannomas, comprising 6–15% of cases.

Symptoms

- Similar to those of vestibular schwannomas: hearing loss, tinnitus, disequilibrium, and vertigo.

Diagnosis

- High-resolution thin MRI and CT scans: presence of a dural tail, invasion of the petrous bone or inner ear structures, and hyperostosis of the petrous bone.

Therapy

- Surgical removal of intrameatal meningiomas should aim at wide excision, including involved dura and bone, to prevent recurrences.

1.25   Paragangliomas of Temporal Bone

Highly vascular, slow-growing neoplasms that develop from paraganglia, which are neurosecretory structures derived from the neural crest.

A. Tympanic paraganglioma (confined to promontory),
B. Jugulotympanic paraganglioma (developed in the jugulo-tympanic region)
   - The most common tumour of the middle ear.
   - Solitary or multicentric (10%, combined with ipsilateral carotid body tumour)
   - In 1–3% of the cases the lesion demonstrates secretory activity (mostly norepinephrine)

Symptoms

- Pulsatile tinnitus
- Hearing loss

   Tympanic Paraganglioma: otalgia, ear fullness, otorrhoea and aural bleeding
   Jugulotympanic Paraganglioma: facial paralysis, lower cranial nerve paralysis (hoarseness, dysphagia)

Diagnosis

- Otoscopy: pulsating retrotympanic vascular mass
- Brown's sign: cessation of pulsation with positive pressure
- MRI: salt and pepper sign in T2 images
- CT: helps to define the extent (Fisch classification)
- Measure of catecholamine levels and 24 h urinary meta-nephrines and vanilmandelic acid.

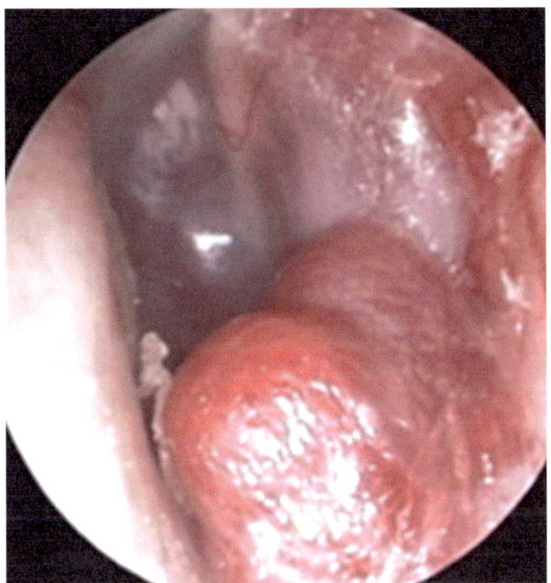

Therapy
Conservative

– No treatment in asymptomatic patients.
– Radiotherapy in older patients and in patients with poor health (to slow or stop the growth)

Surgical

– Transcanal approach: class A (lesion limited to middle ear cavity)
– Mastoid extended facial recess approach: class B (limited to tympano-mastoid area)
– Infratemporal fossa approach with rerouting the facial nerve: C and D (C: involving infralabyrinthine compartment and extending into petrous apoex D: intracranial extension)
– Two stage operation
– Additional treatment modality: Embolization

1.26   Petrous Bone Cholesteatoma

Epidermoid cysts, which have developed in the petrous portion of the temporal bone.

- Congenital: epithelial remnants
- Acquired: deep ingrowths of an epitympanic cholesteatoma

Classification by Sanna: supralabyrinthine, infralabyrinthine, massive labyrinthine, infralabyrinthine–apical, and apical.

Symptoms

- Hearing loss
- Vertigo
- Tinnitus
- Otorrhoea
- Progressive facial paralysis

Diagnosis

- Otoscopy
- Audiometry
- CT: demonstrates bone erosion
- MRI: key examination to demonstrate dura invasion and to differentiate CC from cholesterol granuloma (low signal intensity on T1 scans and high signal intensity on T2).

Therapy
Surgical

The choice of the best surgical approach is based on the location and extent of the lesion, hearing, preoperative facial nerve paralysis, and anatomic position of the internal carotid artery and jugular bulb.
- Marsupialization of the cavity: small infralabyrinthine

- Middle fossa approach: small supralabyrinthine with good hearing
- Modified transcochlear approach: in most cases.

1.27 Petrous Apex Cholesterol Granuloma

Benign cystic lesions that can occur at the petrous apex because of an inflammatory reaction to the byproducts of eroded marrow cavities secondary to chronic obstruction of air cells within the petrous apex.

Symptoms

- CHL (Eustachian tube obstruction)
- SNHL, vestibular abnormalities (compression of IAC)
- Diplopia (compression of VI)
- Facial hypaesthesia (compression of V)

Diagnosis

- CT: visualizes a well shaped enlargement of the apical cell, the bony destruction and relationship to vital structures
- MRI: hyperintense signals on T1 and T2 sequences
- ↑T1, ↑T2

Therapy
Conservative

- Periodic imaging: in asypromatic patients.

Surgery

- Drainage procedures of the petrous apex: infra-labyrintine or infra-cochlear lesion
- Transotic approach: extensive lesion with dead ear

1.28   Zoster Oticus (Ramsay Hunt Syndrome)

Viral infection of the inner, middle, and external ear characterized by:

1. rapid onset of facial nerve palsy
2. severe otalgia
3. ipsilateral vesicular lesions on the auricle and the EAC.

Pathogen: **Varicella zoster virus**

- The virus lies dormant in the geniculate ganglion and is reactivated in times of stress or immunosuppression.

Symptoms

- Facial palsy, burning earache, vesicular lesions
- SNHL, hyperacusis
- Vertigo
- Facial pain (V)
- Pain in pharynx (IX and X)

Diagnosis

Herpes zoster oticus is primarily a clinical diagnosis.
- Inspection/Otomicroscopy: Vesicles
- Nystagmus towards the affected ear, later towards the opposite direction
- Audiometric: SNHL

Therapy
Conservative

- Analgesics
- Local treatment of vesicles with acyslovir cream
- Antiviral agents: Acyclovir
- Coricosteroids: Prednisolone

Surgery

- Golden weight implant in the upper eyelid.
- Hypoglossal-facial anastomosis

- →Prognosis: Incomplete recovery is frequent, worse prognosis than Bell palsy

1.29   Labyrinthitis

Serous or purulent inflammation of the labyrinth caused by bacteria or viruses.

Route of infection:
(1) otogenic, (2) meningogenic, (3) haematogenic

Viral Labyrinthitis

- Otogenic: during the course of a viral infection of URT including the middle ear (picornavirus, influenza/parainfluenza virus, respiratory syncytial virus)
- Meningogenic: during the course of mumps, measles or parainfluenza meningitis. Route of infection are the IAC and the cochlear aqueduct.

Symptoms

- Otogenic: serous effusion of the middle ear, vestibular disturbances, mixed or SNHL, tinnitus, NO earache.
- Meningogenic: clinical signs of meningitis are fatigue, vomiting, headache, stiff neck, fever and unilateral or bilateral deafness.

Bacterial or Purulent Labyrinthitis

- May be secondary to AOM or purulent meningitis [can be a complication of cholesteatoma, spontaneous or acquired labyrinth fistula or may occur in malformations of the cochlea with enlarged perilymphatic spaces (Mondinidysplasia)]

Routes of infection:
In AOM through the oval and round W
Purulent labyrinthitis is frequently followed by meningitis as the microorganisms gain access to the subarachnoid space through the cochlea aqueduct or internal auditory canal.

<u>Complications of Otogenic Bacterial Labyrinthitis</u>: Meningitis, encephalitis, brain abscess, complete deafness, lethal outcome.

<u>Causative agents</u>

Otogenic: pneumococci, Haemophilus influenzae, Streptococcus (A), Escherichia coli and Klebsiella pneumoniae.

Meningogenic: meningococci, pneumococci and Hemophilus influenzae type B.

Symptoms

- Otogenic: severe vertigo with nystagmus, vomiting, high fever. It invariably results in complete HL.
- Meningogenic: classic symptoms of meningitis, severe vertigo with nystagmus, vomiting, unior bilateral, often fluctuating hearing loss or complete deafness. Postinflammatory rapid ossification of the cochlear fluid spaces.

Haematogenic Labyrinthitis
Diagnosis

- Otoscopy: serous or purulent AOM, Pulsating TM, cholesteatoma, bone fracture
- Hearing examination: mixed or pure SNHL
- Frenzel glasses: nystagmus towards the affected ear, later towards the opposite direction.
- H-R "emergency" CT

Microbiology

- Culture taken from the purulent ear secretion
- Blood cell differentiation, blood sedimentation rate
- CSF diagnostics: cell count, protein and sugar elevation, culture taken from the CSF

Therapy
Conservative

<u>Viral</u>

- Glucocorticoids
- Treatment of rhinogenic infection
- Vestibular suppressants
- Antibiotics

<u>Bacterial</u>

- Antibiotics
- Vestibular suppressants

Surgical

- Myringotomy with ventilation tube
- Mastoidectomy
- Labyrinthectomy

1.30   Labyrinthine Concussion

Microinjuries of the inner ear caused by a blunt head trauma.

- Lateral trauma affects the opposite ear (countercoup injury).
- Occipital trauma affects both sides.

Symptoms

- SNHL
- Vertigo
- Tinnitus

Complications

- Luxation of the ossicles
- Progressive SNHL
- Long lasting vertigo
- Perilymphatic fistula
- Subdural bleeding
- Post-traumatic endolymphatic hydrops
- Postconcussion disequilibrium syndrome

Diagnosis

- History
- Inspection
- Otoscopy
- Hearing exam

- Frenzel glasses
- CT scan

Therapy
Conservative
- antioedematous

Surgical

- Reconstruction of the ossicular chain

1.31   Otoliquorrhoea—Otorhinoliquorrhoea

> Abnormal communication between subarachnoid space and middle ear cavity.

Otoliquorrhoea: Outflow of CSF into the EAC through a TM perforation
Otorhinoliquorrhoea: CSF drains into the nose through the Eustachean tube

A. <u>Congenital</u>

Tegmen tympani or tegmenantri defects, Fallopian canal defect
Patent cochlear aqueduct

B. <u>Acquired</u>

Posttraumatic
Postoperative
Symptoms

1. TM perforation: watery pulsating secretion.
2. Intact TM: clear fluid behind the TM, outflow of watery fluid from the nose,

Sensation of salty fluid in the mouth

Diagnosis

- Otoscopy
- Inspection of oral cavity: leak along the posterior wall of pharynx

- Queckenstedt's sign: rise in CSF pressure by compressing the veins in the neck
- HR CT scan
- MRI to prove herniated brain tissue within the temporal bone
- Laboratory tests (glucose/protein content, $\beta 2$ transferrin)
- Intrathecalfluoroscein

Therapy
Conservative

- Rest in bed with elevated head
- Diuretics
- Antibiotics
- Never occlude EAC
- Continuous lumbar CSF drainage

Surgical

- When CSF fistulas do not heal spontaneously

1.32   Perilymphatic Fistula

Abnormal communication between perilymphatic space and middle ear.

Mechanisms of trauma

1. Surgical trauma (stapedectomy)
2. Trauma (temporal bone fracture, barotrauma)
3. Spontaneous
4. Physical exertion

Symptoms

- Sudden or progressive sensorineural hearing loss/vertigo/ tinnitus, may fluctuate
- Episodic vertigo
- Positional vertigo
- Motion intolerance

- Occasional disequilibrium
- may be associated with a positive Hennebert's sign, Tullio's phenomenon, or fistula test

Diagnosis

- Positive fistula sign
- Electrocochleography (ECoG): Increased SP:AP ratios
- CT: may show pneumolabyrinth or middle ear anomalies
- Exploratory tympanotomy: to confirm the diagnosis

Therapy
Conservative

- Bed rest with head elevation
- Laxatives
- Monitoring of both hearing and vestibular function

Surgical

- Exploration of middle ear if hearing loss worsens or vestibular symptoms persist. Plugging of the affected site. Consider plugging both oval and round windows even if no fistula is observed.

1.33   Superior Semicircular Canal Dehiscence Syndrome (SCDS)

> Abnormal communication between middle cranial fossa and superior SCC, creating a third mobile window.

Symptoms

- Vertigo during loud sound (Tullio phenomenon), pressure applied to ear (Hennebert sign), straining (nose pinch or glottis Valsava).
- Abnormally sensitive bone conducted hearing (better than 0 dB thresholds) "can hear my eyes move"
- Pulsatile tinnitus
- Autophony

Diagnosis

- Audiogram: CHL, can be due to suprathreshold bone conduction
- Temporal bone HR-CT scan (0.5 mm slice) [CT may over-diagnose (false positive) or overestimate the size of the dehiscence]
- cervical VEMP and ocular VEMP: decreased thresholds

Therapy

- Surgical plugging of affected SCC.

1.34   Sudden Sensorineural Hearing Loss

Hearing loss of at least 30 dB in at least three frequencies occurring within 3 days.

- Unknown etiology, possible viral or vascular (ischemic) cause.

Symptoms

- Hearing loss
- Vertigo
- Tinnitus

Diagnosis

- Audiogram
- MRI: to rule out vestibular schwannoma (incidence in general population 2/100,000, but as high as 4% in sudden sensorineural hearing loss patients)

Therapy

- Steroids: most recent clinical practice guidelines recommend oral or intratympanic steroids as first line
    - Oral prednisone typically given at 1 mg/kg/day (up to 60 mg) for 7–14 days, then taper

- Intratympanic dexamethasone: can be given alone, as adjunct to oral steroids, or if oral steroid contraindication
- Hyperbaric oxygen: may offer as initial therapy
- Antivirals: not recommended in most recent guidelines

1.35   Benign Paroxysmal Positioning Vertigo

An inner ear disorder that causes brief episodes of vertigo. It is triggered by specific head movements.

<u>Pathophysiology</u>: canalolithiasis or cupulolithiasis
<u>Aetiology</u>: idiopathic, in older age, after head trauma, vestibular neuritis or virtually any inner ear insult.

- The most common cause of vertigo.

  In 96% of cases the posterior vertical canal is concerned,
  Lateral 3%
  Anterior vertical 1%

Symptoms

- Vertigo attacks that last 10–60 s.
- Vertigo is induced by certain head movements.
- No other otological symptoms

Diagnosis

- Dix-Hallpike manoeuvre: turn the patient head 45° towards the left or right side. Then bring the patient from sitting to supine position with head hanging; if present, patient will have vertical (upward) torsional nystagmus.
- Nystagmus begins after several seconds (latency), lasts less than 1 min, is fatiguable, does not change direction BBPV of PV canal.

Therapy

A. Spontaneous resolution in most cases.
B. Liberatory manoeuvres of Semont or Epley (to bring the free-floating otoliths from the semicircular canals to the utricle using gravity).

BPPV of lateral canal
– Barbecue rotation or Brandt-Daroff exercises

C. Surgical treatment (in rare cases with symptoms refractory to repositioning maneuvers)
   – Singular neurectomy
   – Occlusion/plugging of affected semicircular canal

1.36   Meniere's Disease

A disorder of the inner ear characterized by recurrent spontaneous attacks of vertigo (min to hours), fluctuating HL (at low frequencies), tinnitus and aural fullness.

→To confirm the diagnosis:

- At least two episodes of vertigo lasting more than 20 min
- SNHL documented audiometrically at least once.
- Ear fullness and/or tinnitus.
  - The attacks increase in severity and frequency
  - They decrease after 5–10 years.

Diagnosis

- History
- Frenzel glasses: Nystagmus beating away from the affected ear
- Electrocochleography: enhancement of summating potential
- Glycerol test: the subject ingesting glycerol or mannitol (dehydrating agents) and observing for a change in symptoms and a measurable change (improvement) in hearing.
- MRI: to exclude retrocochlear lesion

Therapy
Conservative

<u>In acute attacks</u>: Bed rest, vestibular suppressants, antiemetics

<u>To prevent attacks</u>: Low salt diet, reduced water intake, avoidance of Caffeine-Alcohol-Tobacco, diuretics, antivirals, steroids, vasoactive drugs.

Semiconservative

– Ventilation tube,
– Chemical labyrinthectomy (gentamycin),
– Bilateral cases → streptomycin im
– It dexamethasone
– It ganciclovir

Surgical

– Endolymphatic sac decompression
– Vestibular nerve transection
– Labyrinthectomy (if hearing is already lost)
– Vestibulotomy
– Tenotomy

1.37   Vestibular Neuritis

Acute, unilateral loss of peripheral vestibular function

Aetiology: current findings point to a viral origin (HSV)

Symptoms

– Sudden appearance of severe vertigo that lasts for some
  days.
  Recovery may last weeks or months.
  NO hearing impairment
  COMP: not seldom (15%) BPPV follows VN (Lindsay-
Hemenway syndrome)

Diagnosis

- Frenzel glasses: strong horizontal-rotary nystagmus beating away from affected side.
- Caloric test proves the hypofunction of the lesioned side

Therapy

- H1 antagonists for no longer than 2 days
- Vestibular rehabilitation speeds recovery (to induce vestibular compensation)
- Corticosteroid treatment for the first 14 days.

1.38   Autoimmune Inner Ear Disease (AIED)

It represents less than 1% of all cases of HL or dizziness.

- The diagnosis may be overlooked because of lack of a specific diagnostic test.
- More common in females.
- The first onset of symptoms occurs between 20 and 50 years.

Symptoms

- Hearing loss: a rapidly progressive, often fluctuating, bilateral SNHL over a period of weeks to months. The progression of hearing loss is too rapid to be diagnosed as presbyacusis and too slow to be sudden SNHL.
- Tinnitus: 25–50% of patients also have tinnitus and aural fullness, which can fluctuate.
- Vertigo and/or imbalance: in up to 50% of patients.
- Occasionally only one ear is affected initially, but bilateral HL occurs in most patients (80%), with symmetric or asymmetric audiometric thresholds.
- Systemic autoimmune disease coexists in up to 20% of patients (systemic lupus erythematosus, rheumatoid arthritis, disseminated vasculitis, Sjögren's syndrome, myasthenia gravis, Hashimoto's thyroiditis, Cogan's syndrome, Behçet's disease, sarcoidosis, Wegener's granulomatosis, colitis ulcerosa, relapsing polychondritis).

Diagnosis

- A prompt diagnosis and treatment has a great impact on the hearing prognosis of patients with AIED.
- The diagnosis is based fundamentally on clinical evaluation and the positive response to corticosteroids
  - Detailed history: Endocrine diseases? Recurrent fever?
  - Physical Examination

Otoscopy: usually normal findings; nevertheless external ear skin and/or cartilage inflammation and/or facial palsy may rarely occur (e.g. relapsing polychondritis), as well as tissue destruction at the level of the TM, middle ear and mastoid (Wegener's granulomatosis).

- Laboratory Studies

Recommended tests are:

- Blood tests for auto-immune disorders: levels of circulating immune complexes, Blood Sedimentation Rate, ANA, rheumatoid factor, complement C1Q, smooth-muscle antibody, TSH and antimicrosomal antibodies, antigliadin antibodies (for celiac disease), HLA testing.
- Blood tests for conditions that resemble autoimmune disorders: fluorescent treponemal antibody absorption test (for syphilis), Lyme titre, HbA1c (for diabetes), HIV (HIV is associated with auditory neuropathy).

D/D

- Bilateral Ménière's disease
- Luetic inner ear disease
- Lyme disease
- Toxoplasmosis
- Treatment with ototoxic drugs (gentamicin, cisplatin)
- Charcot–Marie–Tooth disease (hereditary neuropathy)
- Large vestibular aqueduct syndrome
- Endocranic hypertension

Therapy

- The most widely used treatment is corticosteroids therapy.
  - Initial dosage regimen is 60 mg or 1 mg/kg per day of prednisone for a month until the audiogram is stable.
  - The dose is then tapered over 8 weeks to 10–20 mg per day, which is maintained for another 6 weeks.
  - Patients often learn the necessary maintenance dose to preserve their hearing, as the disease activity often waxes and vanishes.
  - In AIED patients, severe adverse reactions have rarely been reported
- In patients that do not respond to steroids or require high doses to control the disease, methotrexate and cyclophosphamide have been tried. These immunosuppressants are associated with considerable toxicity.

Prognosis
If not treated, the inner ear inflammation progresses to severe irreversible damage within 3 months of onset (and often much more quickly). On the other hand, steroid responsiveness is high and with prompt treatment the hearing loss may be reversible. Nevertheless, several patients become steroid dependent.

1.39 Tinnitus

- Objective tinnitus (relatively seldom): Patients notice a real existent endogenous acoustic source originating in middle ear, Eust. tube, soft palate or extra-cranialor intra-cranial vessels.

  Due to spasm of middle ear muscles, myoclonus of soft palate, respiratory noise and breath (patent Eust. tube), or pulsatile noise (due to intracranial hypertension, glomustumor, angioma, aneurysm, AV fistula, stenosis or thrombosis of extra- or intra-cranial vessels, systemic rheological diseases)

- Subjective tinnitus: it is exclusively perceived by the patient. Intermittent or continuous whistling or fizzling, in broad-band or narrowband noise, hum, ping or ringing or even in pure tones of various frequency, intensity and duration. It emerges from deficient neuronal plasticity within the central auditory system triggered by an auditory input failure.

<u>Epidiomiology</u>
Grade I (35–37%): notice tinnitus in silent environment
Grade II (44–51%): tinnitus masked by moderate noise.
Grade III (14–17%):
Perceived even in a loud environment.
<u>Etiology</u>
Subjective tinnitus is a symptom of any diseases of the peripheral or central auditory system:
In 32% caused by noise-induced damage of the inner ear;
In 12% by acute acoustic trauma;
In 8–10% by ISSNHL;
In 8% by Meniere's d;
In 7% presbyacousis;
In 6% labyrinthitis;
In 4% chronic otitis m
In 2–3% otosclerosis;
In 1% vestibular schwannoma.

Diagnosis

1. History
   - Type/character of tinnitus: unilateral, bilateral; intermittent or continuous; frequency; masking level by environmental noise (grade I–III)
   - Visual analogue scale (range from 1 to 10) concerning loudness/annoyance.
   - Onset and duration
   - Potential causal relationship and trigger mechanisms
   - Associated hearing problems, hyperacusis or phonophobia
   - Vestibular complains

- History of orl diseases and surgery
- History of head trauma or other accidents.
- History of internal, neurological, psychiatric or psycho-somatic or orthopaedic diseases.
- Alleviating or amplifying circumstances.
- Tinnitus-associated complaints (sleep disturbance, concentration problems, psycho-emotional and psychosocial problems)
- Profession
- Recreational activities
2. Otoscopy
3. Compression-decompression test using the Politzer balloon.
4. Tympanometry and stapedial reflex.
5. Pure tone audiogram
6. Audiometric tinnitus measurement (frequency matching, intensity, minimal masking level, residual inhibition)
7. Auditory evoked brainstem responses.

Additional

- Rhinoscopy
- Posterior rhinoscopy
- Pharyngoscopy
- Hypopharyngoscopy and laryngoscopy
- Frenzel glasses
- Speech audiometry
- Transitory evoked otoacoustic emissions
- Distortion products of otoacoustic emissions
- Auditory evoked cortical responses.
- Electrocochleography
- Cerebral MRI (in case of pathological ABR or in case of a suspected intracranial disease)
- CT scan of temporal bone (in case of chronic otitis media, mastoiditis, cholesteatoma, head trauma).
- Doppler sonography of extracranial and intracranial vessels (if necessary angio-MRI).

Therapy
Objective Tinnitus

Directed therapy:

- Spasms of the middle ear muscles → myringotomy and insertion of a grommet or transaction of the tensor tympanic muscle or stapedial tendon.
- Myoclonus of soft palate muscles → injection of botulinum toxin.
- Patulous Eustachean tube: myringotomy and insertion of a ventilation tube, paraffin or gelfoam or calcium hydroxylapatite injection at Eustachian tube orifice
- Intracranial hypertension: it may require neuro-surgery in selected cases.
- Angioma, aneurysm, arteriovenous fistula, stenosis, thrombosis of extracranial or intracranial vessels, systemic rheological diseases (hypeglobulinemia or anaemia): these conditions should be treated by the angiologist and vascular surgeons.

Subjective Tinnitus

1. Acute stage (less than 3 months duration)

    - Prednisolone iv on 3 consecutive days. In case of partial or no remission, prednisolone treatment should be continued po for 16 days (+proton pump inhibitors).
    - In case of severe HL, additional iv infusion therapy with hyperosmotic hydrophilic haemodilutive plasma-expanding agent, such as hydroxyethyl starch
    - In case of contraindications for haemodilution, another haemorhoelogical active drug such as pentoxiphylline
    - If this initial therapy is not effective (>25%), hyperbaric oxygenation therapy should be started as soon as possible.

2. Subacute stage (duration of more than 3 months up to 1 year) and chronic stage (duration of more than 1 year).
   - Compensation of the remaining HL using Hearing Aids.
   - Active listening to music of someone's own choice and/ or to audiobooks.
   - Neurofeedback training.

1.40   Ototoxicity

Certain pharmacological agents can cause toxicity of the vestibular (balance) or cochlear (hearing) systems of the inner ear.

Ototoxic medications

- Aminoglycosides (gentamicin and streptomycin more vestibulotoxic; kanamycin, amikacinmore cochleotoxic)
- Macrolide antibiotics
- Loop diuretics
- Salicylates
- Quinines
- Chemotherapy agents

Symptoms

- High pitched tinnitus (earliest sign)
- Oscillopsia, ataxia
- Hearing loss (initially the HL affects high frq)
- Nausea
- Dizziness

Diagnosis

- Audiometry: Sensorineural hearing loss
- Electronystagmography: bilateral caloric weakness
  - Audiometric monitoring of risk patients while using ototoxic medications:

- Establish baseline hearing level
- Repeat test every 2 days
- Monitoring of the status of cochlea with OAEs

Treatment

- Discontinue or change medication
- Antioxidant therapy
- Prophylactic treatment (aspirin)
- Adjustment of doses in patients with decreased renal function

1.41   Presbyacusis

> Progressive symmetric sensorineural hearing loss associated with aging, begins in high frequencies.

Starting in fifth decay.
Pathophysiology: Degeneration of hair cells, cochlear neurons, stria vascularis, cochlear n, central auditory pathway

Symptoms

- HL in high frequencies
- Reduced speech comprehension in ambient noise (party effect)
- COMP: psychosocial isolation

Diagnosis

- History (professional and recreational sound exposure)
- Tone audiometry
- Speech audiogram

Therapy

- Binaural hearing aids
- Phone amplifier
- Resocialization

1.42   Occupational Hearing Loss

Bilateral, mostly symmetric SNHL following intermittent exposure to broadband and/or impulse sound with an intensity above 80–85 dB(A) and a daily exposure of 6–8 h (work shift) over many years.

Symptoms

- Gradual deterioration of hearing
- Because of extensive recruitment, this progressive binaural HL leads to an important communication problem in noisy environments (conversation of multiple persons, theatre, restaurant).
- A pronounced hyperacusis is common.
- Tinnitus is found in 70% of patients.

Diagnosis

- Detailed history
- Complete ENT examination
- Tone audiogram
- Speech audiogram

Therapy

- There is no treatment available to reverse the effects of the disease.
- Hearing aids
- Avoidance of noise or use of ear protection when needed.

1.43   Acute Acoustic Trauma

Broadband sound exposure with an intensity above 100 dB(A) SPL peak equivalent for minutes to hours.

Symptoms

- Sensorineural hearing loss
- A pronounced hyperacusisis common.
- Tinnitus is found in 70% of patients.

Diagnosis

Audiogram
Therapy
There is no treatment available to reverse the effects of
the disease.

1.44   Migraine Associated Vertigo

Variety of dizziness that is associated with migraine
headaches.

- Episodic vertigo occurs in 25–35% of migraine patients;
  most common in women
- Patients may have personal or family history of migraine

Subtypes

- Basilar migraine: patients have two or more symptoms
  (vertigo, tinnitus, hearing loss, ataxia, dysarthria, visual
  symptoms, diplopia, parethesias, paresis, decreased consciousness) followed by a throbbing Headache.
- Benign positioning vertigo of childhood: episodic vertigo
  in children lasting minutes–hours, may progress to
  migraine, strong migraine family history.
- Vestibular: episodic vertigo, constant imbalance,
  movement-associated disequilibrium, lightheadedness
- Headache may occur before, during, or not at all; may have
  photophobia, phonophobia, visual aura
- Motion intolerance, sensitivity to complex visual stimuli
- Hearing loss uncommon, may have unilateral or bilateral
  tinnitus

Diagnosis

- No specific diagnostic tests.
- The diagnosis is based on clinical history, or when the history is unclear, on the therapeutic response to treatment.
- Electronystagmography: normal

Therapy

- Acute phase: triptan, antiemetic medications
- Prophylactic medications: nortriptyline, verapamil, propranolol, topiramate;
- Diet: avoid migraine triggers (MSG, alcohol, aged cheese, chocolate, aspartame)
- Get regular sleep and meals

1.45   Idiopathic Facial Palsy

Acute onset of facial paralysis without detectable cause.

- the most common cause of unilateral facial weakness.
- Unclear cause (viral etiology suspected-reactivation of HSV type 1 in the geniculate ganglion).

Symptoms

- The palsy ranges from weakness of facial movements to a "lifeless" facial drooping on one side.
- Difficulty in eye closure, face twitching, saliva drooling (due to the droopy corner of mouth), dry eye or mouth, taste changes and sometimes hyperacousis and dysaesthesia on the affected side.

Complications

- Disfigurement
- Difficulty with eating, drinking and speaking,
- Dry eye with corneal ulcers and keratitis due to lagophthalmus

– Chronic spasm of face muscles or eyelids
– Taste abnormalities
– Synkinesis (abnormal reinnervation of facial muscles resulting in tears when laughing or inappropriate salivation).

Diagnosis

- History: time and type of onset (slow or rapid), first time or recurrent, additional symptoms (neurological, hearing, vertigo, taste, pain).
- Inspection:
  - Classification according to House and Brackmann;
  - Vesicles (Ramsay Hunt S.).
  - Bell's phenomenon (physiological elevation of the globes when lids are closed) becomes visible owing to incomplete lid closure.
  - Note that peripheral facial palsy includes palsy of the forehead of the affected side.
  - Complete cranial nerve examination. Other neurological signs?
- Palpation: parotid gland (tumour?), dysaesthesia auricle (Ramsay Hunt syndrome?).
- Micro-otoscopy: effusions? cholesteatoma? vesicles? Normal EAC and TM in Bell's palsy.
- Hearing tests: tuning fork, audiogram, tympanogram, stapedial reflexes.

<u>Additional Diagnostic Procedures</u>

1. U/S of parotid gland: to exclude a parotid gland tumor.
2. Electrophysiological evaluation [Electroneuronography (ENOG), electromyography (EMG)]: important for quantification of innervation and reinnervation, prognosis and decision making for surgical intervention.
   EMG results have prognostic value 10–12 days after the onset of facial palsy.
3. Topognostic of facial nerve palsy
   - Tear test (Schirmer test): reduced tear production if palsy is at or proximal to the geniculate ganglion (greater petrosal nerve).

   – Stapedial reflexes: elevated threshold or absence if the lesion is located in or proximal to the tympanic segment of the facial nerve.
   – Evaluation of the taste sense: loss of taste of the anterior two thirds of the lateral tongue shows a loss of function of the chorda tympani and indicates damage proximal to the second genu.
      Note that if all of these tests result in normal findings, the lesion must be distal to the tympanic segment of the facial nerve (mastoid or extracranial segment).

4. Liquor diagnostics: always with synchronous or metachronous bilateral facial palsy (borreliosis? Multiple sclerosis?).
5. Differential blood count, glucose and HbA1c, C-reactive protein, erythrocyte sedimentation rate.
6. Serologic tests for HSV type 1, early summer meningoencephalitis virus, influenza virus, Borrelia burgdorferi and HIV.
7. Balance tests: electronystagmography.
8. Brainstem evoked response audiometry: vestibular schwannoma?
9. HR CT (recommended after trauma): fracture: destructive process, mastoiditis, cholesteatoma?
10. MRI with contrast (if neurotological symptoms are present): evaluates full course of facial nerve (brain, cerebello-pontine angle, internal auditory canal, and parotid gland).

Therapy

1. If the palsy is incomplete and not worsening → medical treatment.
   The patient is clinically observed until total recovery (HB 1).
2. If the palsy is complete but the EMG pattern is favourable, or if daily ENOGs elicit less than an 85% denervation rate → → medical treatment and close follow up.
3. If the palsy is complete and ENOG pattern is unfavourable (90% denervation rate) or if the survey of an initially benign looking Bell's palsy demonstrates a clear clinical

and electrical deterioration $\rightarrow$ $\rightarrow$ surgical decompression of the nerve during the first 3 weeks after onset.

Conservative Therapy

1. Corticosteroids: iv for 3 days. Can be continued orally for several days.
2. Antiviral drug: acyclovir(5×800 mg/day orally).

A combined therapy has better outcome than therapy with corticoids alone.

3. Eye Care

- lubricating eye drops or eye ointments protect the eye.
- An eye patch during sleep.
    - If the patient is referred late (after 3 weeks), the usefulness of any medication is to be discussed.
    - If no recovery at all is observed 6 months after onset, going against the natural evolution of the disease, the diagnosis of Bell's palsy must be reconsidered.

A full MRI and CT scan workup, searching for intrinsic tumors of the nerve, must be performed and surgical exploration of the nerve could be considered.

Surgical therapy

- The aim of the surgery is to decompress the probably swollen nerve by opening the Fallopian canal at the level of the geniculate ganglion and labyrinthine portion to the meatal foramen, thus avoiding total denervation and its associated sequelae (synkinesis, hemifacial spasm; HB 3–4).
- Confirmation of the poor prognosis with EMG (more reliable than with ENOG alone), and realization of a MRI scan are two prerequisites.
- With recurrent paresis, total nerve decompression is a treatment option. If done, it should be performed within 3 weeks to be effective. However, decompression surgery is controversial and has not been shown to routinely benefit patients with Bell's palsy.

<u>Additional Useful Surgical Procedures</u>

– Surgical eye protection (tarsorrhaphia, eyelid gold or titanium inlay).
– Facial reanimation after total palsy: by anastomosis of hypoglossal and facial nerves or with regional muscle transposition (e.g. temporalis transposition).
– Prognosis: the natural evolution of the disease leads 4/5 patients to total or near total recovery (HB 1–2) within some weeks.

1.46   Traumatic Facial Palsy

Facial paralysis resulting from trauma to the nerve in the temporal bone, internal auditory canal or cerebellopontine angle.

<u>Aetiology</u>: Blunt, open, ballistic, or iatrogenic trauma.

<u>Mechanism of injury</u>:

– Immediate onset (direct mechanism)
– Delayed onset (indirect mechanism)

Symptoms

– Facial weakness can be partial or total, immediate or delayed.
– Symptoms depend on the level of the trauma: hypoaesthesia of the Ramsay Hunt area, dry eye due to lacrimal flow defect and ipsilateral hemitongue taste sensation deficit.

Complications
  Conjunctivitis, keratitis, eyeball infections and visual sequelae. Severe aesthetic and functional sequelae.

Diagnosis

1. History of the palsy with regard to the trauma: immediate or delayed.
2. Facial nerve motor function evaluation: House and Brackmann (HB) grading system.
3. Complete otological and neurological workup.
4. A standard audiogram with stapedial reflex measurement is obtained as early as possible.
5. Cranial nerves examination.
6. Eye examination: look for dry eye.
7. HR CT scan (axial and coronal planes): to differentiate transverse translabyrinthine fractures (20%), mainly responsible for lesions to the tympanic portion of the nerve or extralabyrinthine fractures (80%), longitudinal or complex, responsible for lesions in the geniculate ganglion area.
8. Electrophysiological assessment:
   - Electroneuronography (ENOG)
   - Electromyography (EMG) and evoked EMG.

Therapy

1. If the palsy is incomplete, delayed or both → medical treatment.
2. If the palsy is complete but the EMG pattern is favourable (neuropraxia), or if ENOG elicits less than 85% of denervation rate → medical treatment and close follow-up.

If during this survey palsy worsens, the ENOG pattern increases or the EMG pattern favours a severe denervation, a surgical exploration of the nerve is proposed.

3. If the Palsy is Total and Immediate→→Surgery

Conservative Treatment

- Corticosteroids: 2 weeks
- Eye care (closure and eye drops)
- Antiviral drug (acyclovir) use is discussed in the case of a secondarily induced facial paralysis (suspicion of herpesvirus reactivation).

- Physiotherapy and rehabilitation technique
- Vasodilators, pentoxyphilline, dextran

1.47   Facial Nerve Schwannoma

A rare encapsulated benign tumor arising from Schwann cells of seventh cranial nerve.

May arise throughout the course of the facial nerve.

<u>Sites of predilection:</u>

1. perigeniculate area
2. horizontal portion
3. vertical portion

Symptoms

- Depends on the location
- Progressive facial weakness
- Conductive HL

Diagnosis

- Preoperative diagnosis is often unclear
    - Palpation of the neck: mass in parotid region
    - Otoscopy: non-pulsating, grey or redishretrotympanic mass.
    - Audiovestibular testing: PT and speech audiometry
    - Electrical facial nerve testing: EMG, ENOG
    - HR CT and MRI

Therapy
Conservative

- No treatment in patients with no alteration of facial function, esp. in elderly
- Radiotherapy in selected cases

Surgical

- Middle fossa approach: for geniculate and IAC lesions and moderate CPA extension with serviceable hearing.
- Translabyrinthine or transotic approaches: For CPA and IAC lesions without serviceable hearing.
- Transmastoid approach: tympanic & vertical lesions.
- Facial nerve grafting: Complete surgical resection inevitably results in severe facial palsy in most cases. Immediate cable grafting with the great auricular or sural nerve.

Further Reading

1. Jahrsdoerfer R. Congenital malformations of the ear. Ann Otolaryngol. 1980;89:348–53.
2. Carfrae MJ, Kesser BW. Malignant otitis externa. Otolaryngol Clin North Am. 2008;41(3):537–49.
3. Konrad HR, Bauer CA. Peripheral vestibular disorders. In: Bailey BJ, editor. Head and neck surgery-otolaryngology. 4th ed. Philadelphia, PA: Lippincott; 2006. p. 2295–302.
4. Eggers SD, Lee DS. Central vestibular disorders. In: Cummings CW, editor. Cummings otolaryngology—head and neck surgery, vol. 4. 4th ed. Philadelphia, PA: Mosby; 2005. p. 178–9.
5. Yuen HW, Bodmer D, Smilsky K, Nedzelski JM, Chen JM. Management of single-sided deafness with the bone-anchored hearing aid. Otolaryngol Head Neck Surg. 2009;141(1):16–23.
6. Kisilevsky VE, Dutt SN, Bailie NA, Halik JJ. Hearing results of 1145 stapedotomies evaluated with Amsterdam hearing evaluation plots. J Laryngol Otol. 2009;123(7):730–6.
7. Houston DM, Miyamoto RT. Effects of early auditory experience on word learning and speech perception in deaf children with cochlear implants: implications for sensitive periods of language development. Otol Neurotol. 2010;31(8):1248–53.
8. Brant JA, Eliades SJ, Ruckenstein MJ. Systematic review of treatments for autoimmune inner ear disease. Otol Neurotol. 2015;36(10):1585–92.
9. Chien WW, Janky K, Minor LB, Carey JP. Superior canal dehiscence size: multivariate assessment of clinical impact. Otol Neurotol. 2012;33(5):810–5.

10. Beyea JA, Agrawal SK, Parnes LS. Recent advances in viral inner ear disorders. Curr Opin Otolaryngol Head Neck Surg. 2012;20(5):404–8.
11. Makeham TP, Croxson GR, Coulson S. Infective causes of facial nerve paralysis. Otol Neurotol. 2007;28(1):100–3.
12. Lesser TH, Dort JC, Simmen DP. Ear, nose and throat manifestations of Lyme disease. J Laryngol Otol. 1990;104(4):301–4.
13. Fujiwara T, Matsuda S, Tanaka J, Hato N. Facial paralysis induced by ear inoculation of herpes simplex virus in rat. Auris Nasus Larynx. 2016;44(1):58–64.
14. Coelho C, Tyler R, Ji H, Rojas-Roncancio E, Witt S, Tao P, Jun HJ, Wang TC, Hansen MR, Gantz BJ. Survey on the effectiveness of dietary supplements to treat tinnitus. Am J Audiol. 2016;25(3):184–205.
15. Dougherty W, Kesser BW. Management of conductive hearing loss in children. Otolaryngol Clin North Am. 2015;48(6):955–74.

Chapter 2
Nose

P. Koltsidopoulos et al., *ENT*,
DOI 10.1007/978-3-319-56330-5_2,
© Springer International Publishing AG 2017

> Type 3: has a depth of 8–16 mm (0.5% of population)
> The type 3 essentially exposes more of the very thin
> cribriform plate to potential damage from trauma,
> tumour erosion, CSF erosion (in benign intracranial
> hypertension) and local nasal surgery or orbital
> decompression 2.

5. <u>Agger nasi air cells</u> are the most anterior ethmoidal air
   cells lying anterolateral and inferior to the frontoeth-
   moidal recess and anterior and above the attachment
   of the middle turbinate. They are located within the
   lacrimal bone and therefore have as lateral relations
   the orbit, the lacrimal sac and the nasolacrimal duct.

2.1 Nasal Dermoid Cyst

> Epithelium-lined cavities filled with keratin, hair folli-
> cles, sweat glands and sebaceous glands.

– They may have an intracranial connection (20–45%).

Symptoms

– Nasal mass or sinus tract in the midline of the nose.
– It can be located anywhere from the glabella to the
  columella.
– Intermittent discharge of sebaceous material or inflammation.
– Hair protruding through a punctum is pathognomonic.

Complications

– Craniofacial deformation
– Local infection
– Intracranial complications

Diagnosis

• Physical examination: Firm and slow growing mass.
• CT: to visualize bony defects of the skull base.
• MRI: to reveal potential intracranial extension

Therapy

– Early surgical intervention is generally recommended, so as to avoid complications.
– Regardless of the surgical approach, complete excision of the cyst and any associated sinus tract is essential.

2.2 Encephalocele

Herniation of cranial contents through a defect in the skull and the facial bones.

Types

1. Meningocele: it contains meninges
2. Meningo-encephalocele: it contains brain matter and meninges
3. Meningo-encephalo-cystocele: it communicates with the ventricles.

It is caused by failure of the neural tube to close completely during fetal development.

Symptoms

– Midline nasal mass
– Facial disfigurement
– Hypertelorism (telecanthus)
– Nasal obstruction
– Respiratory distress

Diagnosis

Endoscopy: soft, compressible masses whose appearance may be confused with nasal polyps.
    CT: to visualize bony defects of the skull base.
    MRI: to detect intracranial extension of the mass.
    NO BIOPSY

Differential diagnosis

– Dermoid cysts

- Mucocele
- Hemangioma
- Glioma
- Malignant neoplasms
- Lacrimal duct cysts

Complications

- CSF leak
- Meningitis
- Intracranial abscess
- Progressive facial deformity

Therapy

- Surgical management is multidisciplinary in nature.
- It can be done in one stage or multiple stages and consists of excision of the encephalocele sac, repair of the bony defect, correction of telecanthus, and correction of associated deformities ("long nose").

2.3   Choanal Atresia

A condition in which the nasal cavity fails to communicate with the nasopharynx because of failure of one or both nares to canalise.

- The atretic plate contains bone (80–90%) or fibrous tissue (10%).
- Unilateral: more common
- Bilateral: commonly associated with other congenital anomalies (CHARGE syndrome).

Symptoms

- Bilateral atresia: asphyxia and attacks of cyanosis (newborns are obligate nasal breathers). It is considered incompatible with life.
- Unilateral atresia: nasal obstruction and nasal discharge (symptoms present later).

Complications

- Bi: hypoxia with suffocation
- Uni: suckling difficulties leading to weight loss.

Diagnosis

- Endoscopic examination with flexible or rigid endoscopes, when feasible.
- CT scan: the axial views help to assess the thickness of the atretic plate, to distinguish between membranous and bony atresia, and to find out the unilateral or bilateral involvement.

Therapy

- Endoscopic choanoplasty: it is the standard treatment and has good results
- Transpalatal technique: risk of damage of palantine vessels and palatal muscles
- Transnasal approach: puncture with dilator

<u>Postoperative complications</u>

- Restenosis of neochoana (due to scar formation)

2.4   Furuncle

> A localized painful area of cellulitis surrounding a hair follicle leading to abscess formation with accumulation of pus and necrotic tissue.

Causative agent: **Staphylococcus aureus**

Complications

- furunculosis: multiple draining sinuses that may develop into ulcers that heal with a visible scar.

Diagnosis

- Clinical inspection

Therapy

- local heat compresses
- elimination of digital manipulation
- topical antibiotic ointments
- systemic antibiotics directed against *S. aureus*

2.5   Atrophic Rhinitis

Chronic disease of nasal mucosa and subjacent bones, leading to abnormally wide nasal cavities.

Primary: colonization by Klebsiella ozaenae
Secondary: caused by aggressive surgery, trauma, cocaine abuse, radiation exposure, granulomatous disease.

Symptoms

- Foul-smelling nasal discharge
- Crusting
- Dryness
- Epistaxis
- Paradoxical subjective sensation of nasal obstruction (abnormal airflow pattern)

Complications

- Septal perforation
- Saddle-nose deformity

Diagnosis

- History
- Physical examination

Therapy

Conservative (first line of treatment)

- Nasal irrigation with crust removal and local antibiotics.

Surgery

- Young's procedure: closure of nostrils by using a circumferential flap of vestibular skin

2.6   Midline Granuloma

A lymphoma of extranodal presentation with highly aggressive clinical course.

- Greater prevalence in Asian and Latin American countries.
- Association of midline granuloma with EBV

Symptoms

- Nasal obstruction
- The tumor is highly invasive locally (it may infiltrate the lateral nasal wall theorbits and the palate.

Diagnosis

- Biopsy

Therapy

- RT or CRT.
- The prognosis of nasal NK/T-cell lymphoma is extremely poor

2.7   Rhinolith

Rhinoliths are believed to be formed by the deposition of magnesium, iron, calcium and phosphorus around a core, which can be an intranasal foreign body or a body material (blood clot, mucus or bone fragment following trauma).

Types

1. Exogenous: if the core is a foreign material (i.e., beads, paper, buttons)
2. Endogenous: if the core is a body material (i.e., teeth, mucous, bone, blood clot).

Symptoms

Small size: no symptoms
Large size: nasal obstruction, persistent foul-smelling, unilateral nasal discharge.

Complications

Sinusitis, perforation of the nasal septum or the hard palate.

Diagnosis

Anterior rhinoscopy: grey irregular masses that feel hard, bony and gritty on probing
Nasal endoscopy
CT scan

Therapy

– Removal of the existing rhinolith, either by anterior rhinoscopy or nasal endoscopy.
– In some cases a lateral rhinotomy has been required.

2.8 Wegener's Granulomatosis

Systemic chronic vasculitis of small and medium vessels, with an autoimmune component.

It may present with (1) pulmonary, (2) URT or (3) renal involvement.

Symptoms

Localized form (25%): Limited to URT.

– Nasal: rhinorrhea, epistaxis, nasal obstruction, diffuse ulceration, crusting, septum perforation, saddle nose deformity.
– Oral: ulcers, gingivitis
– Laryngeal: hoarseness (laryngeal edema and ulceration), stridor (subglottic stenosis).
– Otologic: otalgia, otorrhea, hearing loss (conductive or sensorineural)
– Ocular: scleritis, conjunctivitis, uveitis.

Disseminated disease

- Upper respiratory tractsymptoms
- Pulmonary involvement: cough, dyspnea, haemoptysis and pleuritic pain.
- Renal involvement.

Diagnosis

- Findings that demonstrate lung (chest x-ray), kidney (urine analysis), or URT involvement (oral or nasal ulcers or discharge).
- c-ANCA: positive blood analysis for cytoplasmic-staining antineutrophil cytoplasmic antibodies
- Biopsy (essential for diagnosis): it should be taken from the involved organ, usually nasal mucosa (multiple turbinate and septum specimens). It often demonstrates no more than non-specific inflammation and necrosis.

Therapy

- High dose steroids for 4 weeks, then tapering.
- Cyclophosphamide for 6–12 months.
- After stabilization of symptoms, maintenance on trimethoprim-sulfamethoxazole
- Management of sinonasal manifestations: Nasal irrigations, topical nasal steroids

2.9 Sarcoidosis

Systemic chronic granulomatous disease of unknown etiology primarily affecting the lungs and the lymph nodes.

Symptoms

- Nasal symptoms: epistaxis, nasal obstruction, nasal pain, crusting, yellow submucosal nodules (granulomas), recurrent sinus infections, anosmia, epiphora, bony erosions.

- Laryngeal: diffuse symmetric enlargement of supraglottic structures, supraglottic or subglottic stenosis.
- Other sites involvement: recurrent bilateral parotid swelling, lacrimal gland swelling.

Diagnosis

- Chest X-rays: to look for pulmonary infiltrates or swollen lymph nodes (lymphadenopathy).
- CT scan: more detailed look at the lungs and lymph nodes in comparison with chest X-ray.
- Pulmonary function tests: to measure how well the lungs are working.
- Bronchoscopy: to inspect the bronchial tubes and to extract a biopsy (a small tissue sample) to look for granulomas and to obtain material to rule out infection.
- Serum/urinary calcium: elevated
- ACE: elevated (83% of patients)

Therapy

- systemic corticosteroids—PO prednisone 10–40 mg/day
- intranasal steroids
- methotrexate
- Spontaneous resolution within 2 years, though 10% progress to pulmonary fibrosis

<u>Heerfordt's disease</u> (uveoparotid disease): variant of sarcoidosis; seen in third to fourth decades; prodrome of fever, malaise, weakness, nausea, night sweats; 5% of patients with parotitis, uveitis, CN paralysis (VII in 50%).

2.10   Systemic Lupus Erythematosis

Autoimmune connective tissue disease, type III hypersensitivity-circulating antibody/antigen/complement immune complex and deposition in basement membrane of dermal-epidermal junction.

- Involves heart, joints, kidneys, skin, blood vessels, nervous system

Symptoms

Head and neck manifestations

- Malar rash (50%)
- Painful oral ulcers (25%)
- Telangectasias
- Septal ulceration/perforation (3–5%)
- Laryngeal/tracheal: true vocal cord thickening/paralysis, cricoarytenoid arthritis, subglottic stenosis
- Acute parotid enlargement (10%)
- Chronic xerostomia
- Cranial neuropathy (15%)

Therapy

Treatment: NSAIDs, antimalarials, glucocorticoids; azathioprine and cyclophosphamide for resistant cases

2.11 Nasal Fracture

Disruption of nasal bone structure, due to trauma.

Sports, falls and assaults are the usual mechanisms of fracture.

Symptoms

- Swelling, deformity, epistaxis, periorbital ecchymosis (suggestive)
- Bony crepitus and nasal segment mobility (diagnostic)
- Epiphora (2%)

Complications

Early:

- Septal hematoma (without drainage it results in abscess formation 6–7 days after trauma, producing necrosis of the septal cartilage).
- Osteomyelitis
- Orbital and intracranial abscesses

- Cavernous sinus thrombosis
- Cerebrospinal fluid leakage
- Meningitis

<u>Delayed</u>

- Saddle nose deformity
- Perforation of septum
- Worsening of septum deviation
- Spurs
- Synechiae
- Internal nasal valve collapse
- Collumerar retraction
- Nasal base widening

Diagnosis

<u>The diagnosis is based mainly on the clinical examination</u>

- Inspection
  - Changes of appearance (deviation and asymmetry), bleeding, watery discharge, changes in nasal breathing and smell.
- Physical examination
  - Palpation: to assess the mobility of nasal bones.
  - Endoscopy: evaluation of internal structures, removal of clotted blood, and assessment of hematoma, mucosal tears and active bleeding is performed.
- Radiography
  - Plain films have up to a high false-positive rate as a result of misinterpretation of normal suture lines.
  - CT is recommended for extensive injuries involving the nasal-orbital-ethmoidal complex.

Therapy

- Treatment of bleeding
  - Conservative: cauterization by silver nitrate, seal with topical materials such as thrombin combined with gelatin foam, fibrin glue, anterior packing (Bleeding from branches of SPA or ethmoid vessels requires anterior-posterior packing).

- Surgical (in refractory cases): direct endoscopic vessel cauterization, ligation, angiography with embolization.
- Reduction

Timing of reduction: Fibrous connective tissue within the fracture line develops 10 days to 2 weeks after injury. Manipulation should be performed before this point. A short delay period of 2–3 days is also recommended to allow for diminishment of swelling.

Type of reduction

– Non-displaced fractures: observation
– Simple injuries (isolated, unilateral with medial displacement): closed nasal reduction. To prevent collapse of the post-reduction framework, nasal packing should be placed for 3–5 days.
– Severe trauma (bilateral, depressed fractures): open approach. Either immediate repair or delayed correction.

2.12 Nasal Septum Deviation

A physical disorder of the nose, involving a displacement of the nasal septum.

Etiology: trauma of nose or midface during birth, in the neonatal period, in childhood or adult life.

Symptoms

– Unilateral or bilateral nasal airway obstruction

Diagnosis

– History: recent nasal trauma, recent nasal surgery, obstructive sleep apnoea.
– Inspection: external dorsal deviation of the columella and caudal septum.
– Rhinoscopy: helpful in diagnosing the location, type and severity of septal deformity.

- Endoscopy: useful in identifying polyps, assessing the severity and extent of posterior septal deviations and bony spurs, and locating areas of septal perforation or mucosal injury. The size of the inferior turbinate should be noted before and after a decongestant spray.
- Cottle's test: lateralising the nasal sidewall with lateral digital pressure on the patient's cheek in order to assess the function of the internal nasal valve.

Therapy

- Septoplasty: aims to straighten the deviated nasal septum.
- Indications of septoplasty before the growth period of nose is finished are very limited.
  - <u>Surgical complications</u>
- Bleeding
- Septalhaematoma
- Septa perforation
- Cosmetic nasal deformities (saddle nose deformity, drooping nasal tip)
- Synechiae
- Hyposmia
- CSF leak (rare, result of damage to the cribriform plate when handling the perpendicular plate of ethmoid, in that case bed rest with elevated thorax to reduce intra-cranial pressure and administration of antibiotics, spontaneous resolution usually occurs).

2.13   Septal Haematoma

Blood collection under the perichondrium of the septum (separates the vascular supply from the cartilage).

- It can result in cartilage necrosis within 3 days.
- One of the most severe early complications of nasal trauma.

Symptoms

- Intense pain
- Complete nasal airway obstruction
- Swelling
- Haematoma of the upper lip and philtrum area.

Therapy

- Drainage through a mucoperichondrial incision.
- Immediate treatment is necessary to prevent long term problems (perforation, saddle-nose deformity, columellar retraction)
- Splints or transtheseptal dissolving sutures are placed to obliterate the potential space and prevent collection.
- Infection involving the septal cartilage requires resection of the cartilage, which is replaced by a septum-like silicon stent. Reconstruction with autologous cartilage is then performed (second stage).

2.14   Saddle Nose Deformity

Characterized by a loss of nasal dorsal height and compromised nasal support structures.

Risk factors

- Groups prone to facial trauma (i.e. boxers),
- History of nasal surgery,
- History of cocaine use,
- Certain familial and ethnic groups.

A. Congenital

- It can be part of individual, syndromic, and ethnic characteristics

B. Acquired

- Traumatic
- Iatrogenic
- Cocaine use
- Wegener's gr.
- Relapsing polychondritis
- Leprosy
- Syphilis

Symptoms

- Nasal obstruction
- Whistling sound heard during nasal airflow
- Nasal crusting

Diagnosis

- History
- Nasal endoscopy

Therapy

- A standard series of photographs should be obtained prior to surgical planning for rhinoplasty.
  - Nasal reconstruction
- Indications for surgery can be functional, aesthetic or most commonly both.
- Contraindications: malignant lesion, chronic or autoimmune diseases, drug abuse, unrealistic expectations, certain professions (boxers and other contact sports)

2.15 Epistaxis

Blood supply of nose

A. ECA:

1. Facial

   (a) superior labial (anterior nasal septum)

2. Internal maxillary

   (a) sphenopalantine   (septum,   inferior/middle turbinates),
   (b) descending palantine (anterior septum)

B. ICA:

1. Posterior ethmoidal
2. Anterior ethmoidal

Types of epistaxis

1. Anterior epistaxis (Kiesselbach area)
2. Posterior epistaxis (Woodruff area)

Causes of epistaxis

A. *Local*: Traumas, iatrogenic, infections, tumors, vascular malformations
B. *Systemic*: Anticoagulant agents, coagulation deficits, hypertension, vasculitis, HHT (Rendu Osler Weber).

Therapy
Conservative

– External pressure to anterior aspect of nose for 10 min
– Nasal cauterization with silver nitrate.
– Nasal packing (anterior with Merocel or posterior with nasal balloons)

Surgical

- Endoscopic bipolar cauterization (SPA, AEA, PEA)
- Selective embolization (polyvinyl alcohol spheres): comp: Blindness, stroke, facial pain, paresthesia
- Arterial ligation (AEA, PEA, IMA, ECA).

2.16 Rendu Osler Weber Syndrome (Hereditary Hemorrhagic Telangiectasia—HHT)

A rare autosomal dominant disorder that affects vessels throughout the body and results in a tendency for bleeding.

Symptoms

- Spontaneous recurrent epistaxis (the most common clinical manifestation)
- Gastrointestinal bleeding
- CNS bleeding (arteriovenous malformations)

Diagnosis

- Multiple telangiectasias of the skin and mucosa

Criteria

1. Epistaxis: spontaneous, recurrent nose bleeds.
2. Telangiectases at characteristic sites (Lips, Oral cavity, Fingers, Nose).
3. Visceral lesions such as:
   Gastrointestinal telangiectasia (with or without bleeding), Pulmonary AVM, Hepatic AVM, Cerebral AVM, Spinal AVM.
4. Family history a first degree relative with HHT according to these criteria.

The HHT diagnosis is:

- Definite ≥3 criteria present.
- Possible: 2 criteria present.
- Unlikely: <2 criteria present.

Therapy

- Recurrent bipolar or laser cautery.
- Septal dermoplasty or Saunder's procedure (skin is transplanted into the nostrils)
- Young's procedure (nostrils are sealed off completely)

2.17   Non-Allergic Rhinitis

Chronic rhinitis with negative testing for IgE-mediated sensitivity to aeroallergens.

Clinical features including obstruction, itching, discharge and sneezing (at least two of them for more than 1 h most days), with negative allergic background (history, skin prick test, serum-specific IgE).

Occupational: exposure to chemicals, biologic aerosols, flour, and latex can lead to symptoms such as sneezing, nasal obstruction and nasal discharge. The symptoms improve when the patient is away from work and worsen throughout the work week. Treatment is based on avoiding the triggering agents (masks, ventilation).

Drug-induced (rhinitis medicamentosa): arises from prolonged use of nasal vasoconstrictors (Oxymetazoline), non-steroidal anti-inflammatory drugs (NSAIDs), Alpha-blockers, Angiotensin-converting enzyme (ACE) inhibitors, Beta-blockers, Cocaine.

- Patients should be advised to use nasal vasoconstrictors for only 1 week.
- To break the cycle of rebound congestion, topical intranasal steroids should be used

Hormonal rhinitis: rhinitis related to metabolic and endocrine conditions, is most commonly associated with high estrogen states (e.g. pregnancy). Rhinitis of pregnancy presents with nasal congestion in the last 6 weeks of pregnancy. There is a complete resolution of symptoms within 2 weeks after delivery.

Rhinitis associated with Physical Factors: a change in temperature, humidity, or barometric pressure or exposure to cold or dry air can cause nasal obstruction and increase of secretions, known as "skier's nose". These triggers are often hard to identify. This type of non-allergic rhinitisis often mistaken for seasonal allergic rhinitis because weather changes occur in close relation to the peak allergy seasons in the spring and fall. Treatment with ipratropium bromide.

Gustatory: spicy foods or alcohol (intranasal atropine)

Atrophic: primary from infection with Klebsiella pneumonia, secondary (from nasal or sinus surgery, trauma, granulomatous disease, or exposure to radiation), progressive atrophy of nasal mucosal, crusting, epistaxis, fetor, hyposmia, and enlargement of the nasal space, although with paradoxical nasal congestion.

Non-allergic Rhinitis Eosinophilic Syndrome: characterized by nasal perennial symptoms. The diagnosis is made when eosinophils account for more than 20% of cells on a nasal smear and allergy testing is negative.

Vasomotor/idiopathic: upper respiratory hyper-resposiveness to non-specific triggers like exposure to strong smells, changes in air temperature or humidity, alcohol ingestion or tobacco smoke. Its diagnosis is based on exclusion of allergy, structural lesions, drug abuse or systemic disease.

Rhinitis and Emotions: stress, sexual arousal

Rhinitis and Gastroesophageal Reflux

Rhinitis and Metabolic Conditions: hypothyroidism, acromegaly

2.18   Allergic Rhinitis

The new ARIA classification of allergic rhinitis is based on symptoms and quality of life parameters.

- Duration of symptoms is subdivided into "intermittent" or "persistent" disease.
- Severity is subdivided into "mild" or "moderate-severe"

Symptoms

- Rhinorrhea,
- Nasal obstruction,
- Nasal itching and sneezing.
- The symptoms are reversible spontaneously or with treatment.

Diagnosis

- History
- Nasal examination: limited information
- Diagnostic tests
    - Skin Prick Test: it gives confirmatory evidence for the diagnosis of a specific allergy.
    - Serum Specific IgE: has value similar to that of skin tests.
    - Allergen Nasal Challenge: useful in the diagnosis of occupational rhinitis.
    - Diagnosis of Asthma: measurement of lung function and confirmation of the reversibility of airflow obstruction are essential in diagnosis of asthma.

Therapy

- Allergen avoidance
- Pharmacological treatment
    - H1 antihistamines: poorly effective against congestion
    - Corticosteroids: the most effective
    - Chromones: intra-ocular are effective, intranasal are not
    - Nasal decongestants: relieve congestion
    - Anticholinergics: block rhinorrhea (atrovent)
    - Leukotriene receptor antagonists (montelukast)
- Specific immunotherapy

2.19   Acute Sinusitis

Defined as a sudden onset of two or more symptoms, one of which should be either nasal blockage/obstruction/congestion or nasal discharge (anterior/posterior nasal drip):

± facial pain/pressure,
± reduction or loss of smell

for <12 weeks.

– The proportion of viral respiratory tract infection (RTIs) that progress to ABRS is relatively small (2%).

<u>Risk factors</u>: Asthma, allergy, cystic fibrosis, suppression of the immune system, smoke exposure, cocaine use
Pathogens: Streptococcus pneumoniae and Haemophilus influenzahaemophilus influenzae and less commonly S. aureus and M. catarrhalis, various streptococci, and a minority have anaerobes such as bacteroides and anaerobic streptococci.

Symptoms

– Diagnostic symptoms
– Minor symptoms: sore throat, dysphonia, and cough, and general symptoms including drowsiness, malaise, and fever

Diagnosis

• Diagnosis is based on the symptoms
• Nasal endoscopy: purulent discharge from the middle meatus, oedema/mucosal obstruction primarily in the middle meatus
• Oral examination: posterior discharge; exclude dental infection.
• Imaging: only in severe/complicated cases. The plain sinus x-ray is not recommended. CT scanning is the modality of

choice for the paranasal sinuses due to optimal display of air bone and soft tissue.
- Samples under endoscopic guidance (good alternative to sinus puncture)
- <u>Differential diagnosis between viral and bacterial rhinosinusitis</u>
  - Acute bacterial rhinosinusitis signs and symptoms are not specific and are difficult to differentiate from viral RTIs
  - Lack of reliable, convenient and practical diagnostic tools.
    Common cold/acute viral rhinosinusits: duration of symptoms for less than 10 days.
    Acute post-viral rhinosinusitis: increase of symptoms after 5 days or persistent symptoms after 10 days with less than 12 weeks duration.
    Acute bacterial rhinosinusitis (ABRS): presence of at least three symptoms/signs of.
- Discoloured discharge (with unilateral predominance) and purulent secretions
- Severe local pain (with unilateral predominance)
- Fever (>38 °C)
- Elevated ESR/CRP
- 'Double sickening' (i.e. a deterioration after an initial milder phase of illness)

Therapy

<u>Goals of therapy</u>

- restore the integrity and function of ostiomeatal complex by reducing inflammation and restoring sinus drainage
- eradicate the bacterial cause of infection
- avoid complications

Conservative treatment
Initial therapeutic stratefy depends on the severity of the disease:

- Mild (viral, common cold): watchful waiting combined with symptomatic therapy (analgetics, saline irrigation, decongestants, steam inhalation, herbal compounds);

- Moderate (postviral): additional topical steroids
- Severe (including bacterial): additional topical steroids, antibiotics
  - First-line: Amoxicillin
  - Second-line (no improvement after 3 days): second generation cephalosporins, macrolides and fluoroquinolones.

Surgical Treatment

- Antral puncture has become rare since the inception of antibiotics.
- Functional endoscopic sinus surgery: in severe or complicated cases.

2.20   Cronic Rhinosinusitis

It is defined as presence of two or more symptoms one of which should be either nasal blockage/obstruction/congestion or nasal discharge (anterior/posterior nasal drip):

- ±facial pain/pressure;
- ±reduction or loss of smell;

for ≥12 weeks

Types

1. Chronic rhinosinusitis without nasal polyps (CRSsNP)
2. Chronic rhinosinusitis with (CRSwNP)

Associated factors: ciliary impairment, allergy, asthma, aspirin sensitivity, immunodeficiencies, genetic factors, biofilms, iatrogenic factors

Inflammatory triggers: bacteria, fungi, allergens, viruses, environmental factors

Symptoms

- Diagnostic symptoms
- Minor symptoms: ear pain, tooth pain, dizziness, halitosis, laryngeal and tracheal irritation, dysphonia, cough, drowsiness, malaise and sleep disturbance,

Diagnosis

- Diagnosis is based mainly on the symptoms
- Nasal endoscopy: oedema/mucosal obstruction primarily in middle meatus, mucopurulent discharge primarily from middle meatus, nasal polyps
- CT scan: mucosal changes within the ostiomeatal complex and/or sinuses
- Biopsy: may be indicated to exclude more sinister and severe conditions such as neoplasia and vasculitides.

Therapy

A. <u>Management for adults without NP</u>

- topical steroids
- nasal saline irrigations
- long term oral antibiotic therapy: esp. if IgE is not elevated
- functional endoscopic sinus surgery

B. <u>Management for adult with NP</u>

- topical steroids
- oral steroids (short course)
- doxycycline
- nasal saline irrigation: for symptomatic relief
- functional endoscopic sinus surgery

2.21   Fungus Ball (Mycetoma)

> Accumulation of non-invasive fungal dense concretions at the level of the paranasal cavities.

It occurs in immuno-competent patients.

<u>Sites of involvement</u>

– maxillary sinus (most common)
– sphenoid sinus

<u>Causative species</u>

Aspergillus Fumigatus (the most common).

Symptoms
Non-specific complaints similar to those of chronic rhinosinusitis.
    Chronic pain (retro-orbital when the sphenoid is involved), purulent rhinorrhea, cough, nasal obstruction and cacosmia.

Diagnosis
Fungus balls are frequently incidental findings on imaging.

Nasal endoscopy:

• Purulent secretions
• Oedema, sometimes with localized polyps
• Fragments of fungus ball

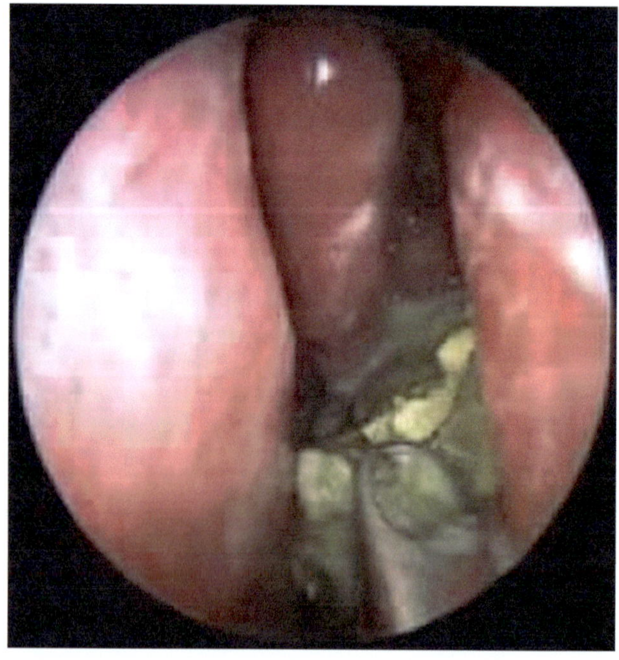

CT:

- Unilateral partial or complete opacication of a single sinus, usually the maxillary sinus.

Bone thickening or bone lysis of the nasomaxillary wall

- Macrocalcifications (pseudometallic foreign body)
- Sometimes bone erosion (pseudo-tumoral image)

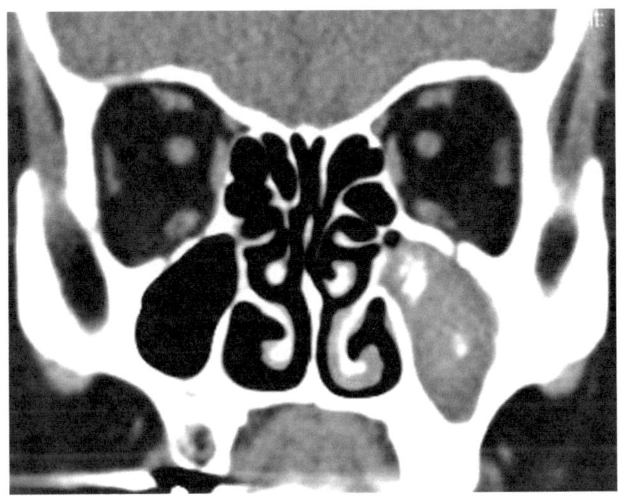

MRI: to differentiate a fungus ball from tumours, or invasive fungal rhinosinusitis (in immunocompromised patients).
   T1: Hypodense signal
   T2: Hypodense signal
   The mucosa has hyperdense signal on *T*2- and post-gadolinium *T*1-weighted sequences.

Therapy
Complete surgical removal of fungus ball. Antifungal therapies are unnecessary.

- The macroscopic aspect of the fungus balls during surgical removal is often highly suggestive: a solid but crumbly, from brown- to black-coloured mass, with thick creamy secretions.

Surgery goals:

1. Complete removal of the fungus ball and secretions while preserving the integrity of the mucosa
2. Recovery of sinus drainage and ventilation
3. Easy endoscopic follow-up

2.22   Allergic Fungal Rhinosinusitis

– The diagnosis of allergic fungal rhinosinusitis (AFS) was developed for patients with recurrent nasal polyps and asthma in mind, but there is still not a clear definition and/or panel of criteria.
– Clearly different from allergic rhinitis with fungus IgE-mediated sensitisation.

Symptoms

– Nasal obstruction
– Nasal discharge
– Sneezing,
– Headache
– Dysosmia.
– Nasal polyposis may be unilateral and may be aggressive, with orbital signs (proptosis, diplopia, visual loss). Asthma is frequent.

Diagnosis

• Inspection: may show cheek and/or palpebral swelling, proptosis, ophthalmoplegia.
• Nasal endoscopy: may be normal or show mucosal oedema, or polyps with or without allergic mucin (thick yellow–green mucus plugs) on one or both sides.
• CT scan: may reveal heterogeneous and serpiginoussinus opacities, with or without pseudo-calcifications and bone lysis on one or both sides.
• Biopsy: allergic mucin with detection ofhyphae, eosino-phils and Charcot-Leyden crystals.

- Mycology: involves identification of various species on mucus fungal culture.
- Serum hypereosinophilia may be present.
- Type I hypersensitivity to fungal species is frequent.
- There may be evidence of asthma.

Therapy

- Still no consensus.
- Large surgical removal of lesions, mainly via endoscopic sinus surgery.
- Postoperative systemic steroids are recommended by most authors for a duration varying from 2 weeks to several months.
- Antifungal agents (local or systemic) are recommended by some authors.

2.23   Invasive Fungal Rhinosinusitis (RS)

Defined by the presence of fungal tissue invasion, detected on pathologic examination.

Clinical forms

1. Acute invasive fungal RS,
2. Indolent invasive fungal sinusitis and chronic invasive fungal sinusitis.

Acute Invasive Fungal RS
In immuno-compromised patients (esp. leukaemia and lymphoma).

- Neutropenia is a key factor (esp. when neutrophils <500/ml).

Other risk factors: long-term steroid therapy, graft-versus-host disease, AIDS, diabetes, radiotherapy, long-term antibiotic therapy and malnutrition.

Mucormycosis (caused mainly by the genera Rhizopus or Absidia) represents a distinct entity, as it is generally met in type I diabetes patients.

Symptoms

Palpebral or cheek swelling.

– Unexplained fever in immunocompromised patients.
– nasal congestion,
– rhinorrhea,
– epistaxis and/or
– headaches.

Diagnosis

Nasal endoscopy: oedema, ulcerations & necrosis with crusts.
   CT/MRI: sinus opacities, bone necrosis and orbital and/or intracranialinvasion.
   Biopsy: fungal elements invading the mucosa, with thrombosis, ischaemia and necrosis.
   Culture: mainly A. fumigatus and Aspergillus flavus.

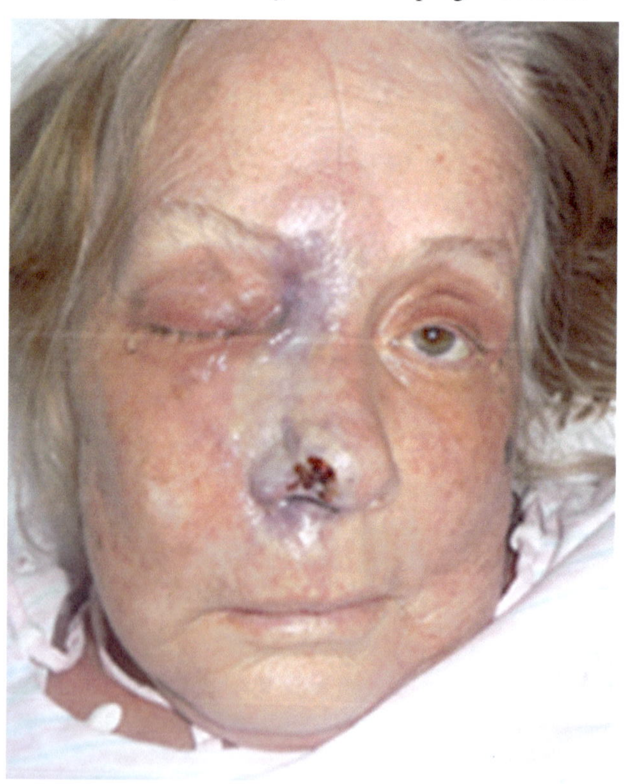

Differential Diagnosis

Other types of rhinosinusitis, infectious (Pseudomonas aeruginosa, tuberculosis, syphilis, rhinoscleroma), inflammatoryor
granulomatous (sarcoidosis, Wegener's disease) may exhibit
vascular or tissue necrosis.

Therapy

1. Amphotericin B
2. Itraconazole (generally recommended after amphotericin
   therapy).
3. Surgical excision of invaded tissues.
   (via an external approach, or in selected cases via an endoscopic approach). Orbital involvement may lead to larger
   excisions.
   In cases of intracranial invasion a combined transcranial
   approach must be discussed.
   – Long follow-up (endoscopy and imaging) is mandatory:
     recurrences may happen in cases of new occurrences of
     neutropenia.
   – Prognosis: a mortality rate of 20–80% in immunocom-
     promised patients is reported.

2.24 Complications of Sinusitis

Classification

A. orbital (60–75%)
B. intracranial (15–20%)
C. osseous (5–10%)

Pathogens

– Children: H influenza
– Adults: staphylococcus, Str. Pneumonia

Orbital (cefuroxime)

– The most common complications of rhinosinusitis
– Associated in order of decreasing frequency with the ethmoid, maxillary, frontal and rarely the sphenoid sinus

- Spread pattern of infection: directly via the thin and often dehiscent lamina papyracea or by veins.
- Orbital complications in children may occur without pain

<u>Chandler's classification</u>:

   I. preseptal cellulitis
  II. orbital cellulitis
 III. subperiosteal abscess
 IV. orbital abscess
  V. cavernous sinus thrombosis

Preseptal cellulitis: involves the tissue anterior to the orbital septum, usually responds to oral antibiotics. It occurs often as a complication of upper respiratory tract infection, dacryocystitis or skin infection and less often sinusitis

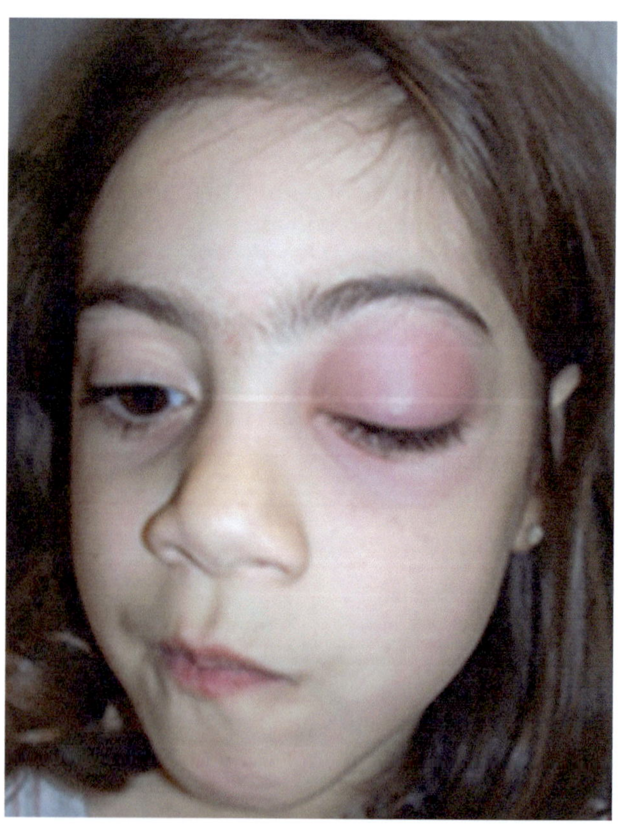

Orbital cellulitis: it presents with conjunctival oedema (chemosis), proptosis, ocular pain and tenderness, restricted and painful movement of the extraocular muscles.

CT scan with i.v. contrast of the sinuses: to exclude intra-orbital or subperiosteal abscess.

It requires aggressive treatment with intravenous antibiotics.

Subperiosteal abscess: pus between periorbita and the sinuses. It presents with oedema, chemosis and proptosis of the eyelid, limitation of ocular motility, diminished visual acuity. CT scan: oedema of the medial rectus muscle, lateralization of the periorbita, and displacement of the globe downward and laterally.

Orbital abscess: abscess contained within the space defined by the ocular muscles. It presents with severe proptosis, complete opthalmoplegia, impaired visual acuity

CT scan: obliteration of the detail of the extraocular muscle and the optic nerve by a confluent mass.

Evidence of an abscess on the CT scan or absence of clinical improvement after 24–48 h of i.v. antibiotics are indications for orbital exploration and drainage. Intravenous antibiotic therapy should cover aerobic and anaerobic pathogens.

Cavernous sinus thrombosis: through orbital v. sepsis. Rare and dramatic complication. Main symptoms: bilateral lid drop, retro-ocular pain, proptosis, complete opthalmoplegia, papilloedema, spiking fevers.

MR venogram: demonstrates absence of venous flow in the affected cavernous sinus.

High-resolution CT scan with contrast: shows filling defects.

Therapy: anticoagulants (controversial), steroids, antibiotics, drainage of the offending sinus (almost always the sphenoid).

Intracranial (frontal, ethmoid, sphenoid)

- They are most often associated with frontal, ethmoidal or sphenoid rhinosinusitis
- Pathogens: Streptococcus and Staphylococcus species and anaerobes
- Two different spread patterns: pathogens, starting can pass through the diploic veins to reach the brain; alternatively, they can reach the intracranial structures by eroding the sinus bones or haematologically

- CT scan with contrast: essential for diagnosis.
- MRI: more sensitive than CT
- Lumbar puncure: if meningitis is suspected
- Therapy: high dose long-term i.v. antibiotic therapy followed by burr hole drainage, craniotomy or image guided aspiration as needed.

Combined drainage of the paranasal sinuses (often the frontal sinus) can be performed endoscopically.

Meningitis: sever headache, high fever, nuchal rigidity (Cefotaxime)

Epidural abscess: often indolent

Subdural abscess: neurologic deficit, seizures

Brain abscess: headache, fever, nausea, vomiting, seizures. (Cefotaxime)

Osseous

- Sinus infection can also extend to the bone producing osteomyelitis and eventually involving the central nervous system.
- The most common osseous complications are osteomyelitis of the maxillary (typically in infancy) or frontal bones.
- Pott's puffy tumor: osteomyelitis of the frontal bone and associated subperiosteal abscess.
- Signs and symptoms of intracranial involvement: high fever, severe headache, meningeal irritation, nausea and vomiting, diplopia, photophobia, papillary oedema, coma and focal neurological signs.
- Contrast- enhanced CT scan confirms the diagnosis.
- Therapy: i.v. broad-spectrum antibiotics and surgical debridement of sequestered bone and drainage.

Diagnosis

- Nasal endoscopy
- White cell count: elevated, unresponsive to treatment
- Ophthalmologic exam: extra-ocular movements, visual acuity
- CT with contrast
- MRI: to identify intracranial extension

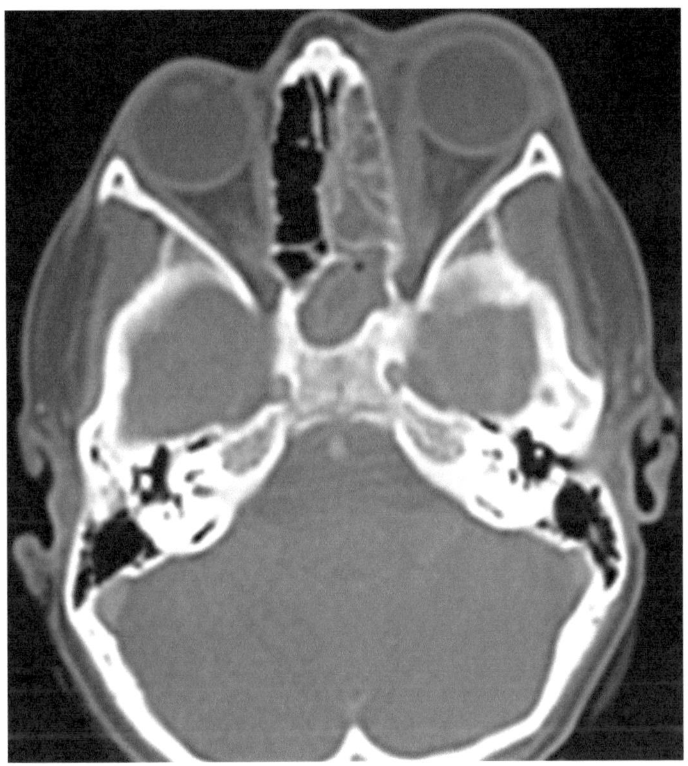

2.25 Paranasal Sinus Mucocele (PSM)

Epithelium-lined cystic masses usually resulting from obstruction of sinus ostia.

- The frontal sinus is most commonly affected followed by the ethmoid sinuses (70–90%).
- The close proximity of PSMs to the orbit and skull base predisposes the patient to significant morbidity.

Symptoms

Symptoms depend on the location of the mucocele:

– Ophthalmologic (most common): proptosis, hypoglobus, diplopia, periorbital swelling, visual compromise and optic neuropathy
– Rhinological
– Neurologic

Diagnosis

– CT: non-enhancing homogenous mass with expansion of bony walls.
– MRI: imaging reveals variable intensity of T1-weighted images and a hyperintense mass on T2-weighted images.

Therapy

– Surgical excision through an open approach or endoscopically.

2.26   Silent Sinus Syndrome (SSS)

Painless enophthalmos associated with chronic maxillary atelectasis with complete or partial opacification of the sinus.

Pathophysiology: Chronic occlusion of the maxillary sinus ostium → resorption of air → → negative pressure → gradual inward bowing of all four of the maxillary walls: roof (orbital floor), medial, posterolateral and anterior walls → orbital volume increases with resultant enophthalmos

Symptoms

– Facial asymmetry
– Enophthalmos
– Hypoglobus

Diagnosis

- CT scan: thinning and retraction of the orbital floor, ipsi-lateral maxillary sinus hypoplasia and opacification, later-alization of the uncinate process resulting in blockage of the ostiomeatal complex and retraction of the posterolat-eral and medial walls of the maxillary sinus.

Therapy

- FESS: enlargement of the maxillary ostium in order to restore normal sinus drainage.
- Once drainage is established, no further volume loss will develop. However, any deformity at the time of surgery will be permanent.
- Repair of the orbital floor with placement of a subperios-teal implant: in patients with diplopia or severe cosmetic deformity.

2.27   Frontal Sinus Trauma

Fracture of the anterior orposterior table of the frontal sinus

- The frontal bone is the strongest component of the cranio-facial skeleton
  Causes: motor vehicle accidents, sports-related injuries, industrial accidents.

Complications

- Frontal sinusitis (caused by a blocked frontal ostium, retained foreign bodies or bony chips)
- CSF leak (when there is an open posterior table fracture with rupture of the dura mater).
- Meningitis
- Brain abscess

- Mucocele (caused by obstruction in the frontal ostium or trapping of respiratory epithelium)
- Mucopyocele

Diagnosis

- Inspection
  - Skin lacerations
  - Asymmetry or depression of the forehead
  - Ecchymoses and/or ecchymosed
- Palpation
  - Pain with pressure
  - Step-off fractures or crepitus
  - Anaesthesia in the supraorbital nerve distribution
- Rhinoscopy
  - Epistaxis
  - Clear rhinorrhea, which is suggestive of a CSFleak (β-trace protein test, β-2 transferrin test, or intrathecal fluorescein).
- CT (axial and coronal views as well as sagittal reconstruction).
- MRI: to exclude brain injuriesor intracranial haematoma

Therapy

- Goals of frontal sinus fracture management
  - Restore function
  - Restore facial contour
  - Avoid complications

A. _Anterior_ table fractures

  - Non-displaced fracture with no involvement of the frontal sinus outflow tract (FSOT): conservative treatment.
  - Minimally displaced fractures: Minimally invasive endoscope-assisted frontalrepair.
  - Significantly displaced fractures with obstruction of the FSOT: Open reduction and internal fixation

B. <u>Posterior table fractures</u>

- Linear or non-dislocated fractures without evidence of CSF leak: conservative treatment
- Minor displaced fractures: Trepanation and transcutaneous endoscopy
- Significantly displaced fractures with obstruction of the FSOT: open approach.
- Total obstruction of the FSOT that cannot be resolved through an endoscopic or open approach: Frontal sinus obliteration (abdominal fat after obstruction of the FSOT by using fascia or a galea-periost flap).

2.28   Fractures of Midface

<u>Classification according to Le Fort</u>

- Le Fort I: The lower alveolar and palatal regions are separated from the upper maxilla in a horizontal plane above the teeth apices and the hard palate. It results in a mobile palate, but a stable upper midface.
  - The fracture line extends through the lateral nasal wall and pyriform aperture, across the maxillary alveolus and antral walls to the pterygoidplates.
  - Result from anterior forces directed at the lower midface.
- Le Fort II: Characterized by a dissociation of the maxilla, the nasal bones, and the nasal septum from the cranial skull and from the lateral midface.
  - The fracture line extends through the nasofrontal suture lines, the lacrimal bones, the inferior orbital rims, across the maxillas at or near thezygomatic-maxillary suture lines, and down through the lateral maxillary sinus walls and through the pterygoid plates.
  - Result from forces applied near the level of the nasal bones

- Le Fort III: The facial skeleton is separated from the cranial skull.
  - Fracture line extends through nasofrontal sutures, the medial orbital walls, through the inferior orbital fissures to the lateral orbital wall at the zygomatic-frontal suture and across the zygomatic-temporal suture.
  - Result from anterior forces directed obliquely to the plane of the vertical buttresses.

Symptoms

- Le Fort I
  - Malocclusion and an anterior open-bite deformity
  - Haematomas and parietal fractures in maxillary sinuses
  - Airway compromise (if palateretrusion is severe).
- Le Fort II
  - Moderate dislocation
  - Midfacial depression, with participation of sphenoid, orbital content, lacrimal ducts (epiphora) and on some occasions, telecanthus or CSF leakage
- Le Fort III
  - Facial tumefaction, haematoma, bleeding, eventually shock, commotion or cerebral contusion, loss of vision secondary to intraorbital haemorrhage or to direct optic nerve lesion
  - Complete craniofacial dislocations, often associated with neurosurgical injuries
  - CSF leakage
  - Significant orbital trauma
  - Loss of vision and multiple fractures of the craniofacial skeleton ("dish face")

Diagnosis

- Inspection
  - Asymmetries of midfacial/frontal region
  - Periorbital ecchymosis
  - Massive tissue swelling or subconjunctival haemorrhage
  - Open bite

- – Lingual/buccal region involvement
  - – Subcutaneous emphysema
  - – Nasal or pharyngeal haemorrhage
- Palpation
  - – Pain with pressure
  - – Abnormal mobility of the palate
  - – Interruption of normal face structures
  - – Steps or tenderness of underlying bony skeleton
  - – Bony crepitation of the midface
  - – Immobility of the jaw in all directions, malocclusion and altered state of teeth
- Pharyngoscopy
  - – Teeth avulsion
  - – Mucosal injuries
  - – Haematomas and ecchymosis (evidence of nonvisible fractures)
- Rhinoscopy
  - – Rhinorrhea
  - – Epistaxis
  - – Septal luxation
  - – Septal haematomas
- Visual examination (open-eye injuries and any cause of visual loss must be repaired in the first 6 h after injury)
  - – Ocular movement
  - – Visual acuity
  - – Pupillary function
  - – Campimetry
- CT scan in three levels
  - – Status of the buttress system
  - – Zygomatic arches
  - – Orbital volume and herniation of orbital contents
- MRI: to rule out cerebral trauma or compression of the optic nerve

Therapy

- Goal: reconstruction of the shape and function of all structures of the midface by open reduction and internal fixation.

- The treatment should be performed when the patient's situation is stable (Breathing, Bleeding, Shock, Brain, Vision, Nutrition)
- Nasogastric nutrition tube: in cases with injuries of the orohypopharynx
- Tracheostomy: when long-term interdental fixation is planned.
- Arch bars and maxilla-mandibular fixation (MMF): in patients with functioning dentition
- Splint or denture containing an arch bar is fixed to the mandible or maxilla, with circum-mandibular wires or drop wires from the pyriform rim or zygomatic bone: in edentulous patients
- In patients with displaced midfacial fractures, a downward and anterior pull by use of the Rowe-Killey forceps will replace the maxilla and restore its normal position.
- Le Fort I: extended sublabial incision
  - A two-point stabilisation at the nasomaxillary and zygomatic-facial buttresses is established. Titanium or polyglycolic/polylactic acid, low-profile mini-plates, or a combination of both, are placed on the anterior buttresses along with (usually) an L-shaped plateon each zygomatic bone onto the maxilla.
- Le Fort II: transconjunctival-lateral canthotomy or subciliary incision
  - If a greater exposure to the nasoethmoidal complex is required, an external Lynch incision or an extended coronal incision may be used.
  - Fixation at the infraorbital rim and the zygomatic-maxillary buttresses
  - If the nasal bones are comminuted, microplates are used to restore nasal contour.
- Le Fort III: the maxilla must be fixed between cranium and mandible.
  - All displaced fractures of the cranial vault and mandible must be restored to provide two stable platforms.
  - Functional elements must be restored (correct orbital volume, adequately restored orbital floor with orbital

contents free of entrapment, patent nasal airway bilaterally and maxillary sinuses that will adequately drain).
  – The lateral orbital rims and the buttresses are fixed with miniplates and the nasal dorsum and infraorbital rims with microplates.
- If rigid fixation is considered stable, the MMF may be removed at the end of the operation or within the first 1–2 weeks after the operation.
- If no stability has yet been achieved, the MMF should be left in place for up to 6–8 weeks.
- <u>Surgical complications</u>
  – Malunion and resultant malocclusion with temporomandibular joint dysfunction and deformity (if reduction is not precise, or if loosening of fixation occurs).
  – Dehiscence-type defects: (because of inadequate closure during surgery, poor oral hygiene, local trauma or excessive motion).
  – Injury to tooth roots from misplaced screw holes
  – CSF leak
  – Epiphora

2.29   Zygomatic-Maxillary Complex Fracture

Any isolated or combined fracture of the malar eminence and/or the zygomatic attachments.

- The second most common facial fracture after nasal bone fractures.

Diagnosis

- Inspection
  – Swelling, haematoma, malar and periorbital ecchymoses and malar depression.
  – Trismus.

- Ophthalmic findings: inferior displacement of lateral canthal tendon, subconjunctival haemorrhage and proptosis;

<u>Acute orbital hematoma</u> <u>may cause loss of vision by compression of ophthalmic artery or optic nerve!</u>

- Palpation
  - Pain on palpation and crepitation from subcutaneous emphysema (which in most cases is caused by blowing the nose)
  - Bony step-off when palpating the infra-orbitalrim, the frontal zygomatic suture line and intraoralin the zygomatic-maxillary buttress
  - Anaesthesia caused by compression of the infraorbital nerve.
- Rhinoscopy
  - Ipsilateral epistaxis
- HR CT (axial and coronal views)
  +Waters view radiograph

Complications

- Diplopia
- Loss of vision
- Lower eyelid malposition (ectropion, entropion)
- Enopthalmos
- Malocclusion

Therapy

- **Conservative therapy**
  - In cases with non-displaced or minimally displaced ZMC fractures and a normal ophthalmologic examination.
- **Surgical therapy**

<u>Indications</u>

1. Facial contour alteration
2. Persistent difficulties in chewing

3. Visual changes caused by muscle entrapment, globe displacement and orbital floor disruptions.

<u>Surgical principles</u>

- Goals of frontal sinus fracture management
  - Restore facial contour
  - Avoid complications
- Surgical approaches (depend on the site of the fracture)
  - Transverse buccal sulcus incision.
  - Upper lid blepharoplasty incision
  - Lateral brow incision
  - Hemicoronal incision.
  - Orbital rim incision
  - Transconjunctival approach
  - Direct percutaneous approach
  - Temporal approach
  - Gillies approach
- Prognosis
  - Long-term prognoses in ZMC fractures are very good.
  - 3–4% have residual facial asymmetry.
  - 7% persistent diplopia.

2.30   Fracture of Orbital Floor (Blow Out)

Fracture of orbital floor without fracture of orbital rim, from blunt trauma to bulbus oculi.

Diagnosis

- History
- Inspection
  - Periorbitaloedema and ecchymoses
  - Subconjunctival haemorrhage
  - Enopthalmos and ptosis of globe

- Periocular air emphysema after nose blowing
- Diplopia
- Reduced ocular motility (limitation of upgaze, down-gaze, or both-entrapment of inferior ocular muscles).
- Palpation
  - Bony step at the lower rim of the orbit
  - Hypoesthesia in the distribution of the infraorbital nerve.
- CT scan with coronal or sagittal views: to evaluate fracture size and extraocular muscle relationships.
- MRI: to evaluate intra-orbital hematoma, dislocated soft tissue masses and optic nerve pathology.

Complications

- Loss of vision (result from globe trauma, injury to the optic nerve, or increased orbital pressure causing a compartment syndrome)
- Permanent diplopia, neuralgia and ocular muscle dysfunction
- Recurrent sinusitis maxillaris

Therapy

- **Conservative therapy**

  - The majority of blowout or other orbital floor fractures do not require surgical intervention.
  - Observation for 5–10 days to allow swelling and orbital hemorrhage to subside.

- **Surgical therapy**

Indications

- Tight entrapment of the inferior rectus muscle causing diplopia.
- Enophthalmos that exceeds 2 mm and is cosmetically unacceptable to the patient (enophthalmos is usually masked by orbital edema immediately after the trauma).

- Large fractures involving at least half of the orbital floor, particularly when associated with large medial wall fractures (determined by CT).
- If there is any evidence of increased intra-orbital pressure or optic nerve lesiona lateral canthotomy with cantholysis is indicated.

<u>Surgical principles</u>

- The ideal time for the repair of blowout fracturesis either immediately or 7–14 days after the injury, when the oedema/haematoma have been resolved.
- Surgical technique
  - Transconjunctival, subciliary, inferior fornix ormid-lower eyelid incision
  - Orbital contents are raised out of the fracture line and supported with a titanium plate, thinned cartilage, bone fragments to be found in loco, resorbable plate or polydioxanone (PDS) plate.
- <u>Postoperative complications</u>
  - Persistent infraorbital nerve dysaesthesia.
  - Persistent diplopia.
  - Enophthalmos can worsen over time (atrophy of the orbital fat can occur).

2.31   Smell Disorders

Types of olfactory disorders

- Anosmia: complete loss of detection and recognition of smell.
- Hyposmia: general decreased sense of smell.
- Hyperosmia: increased sensitivity to all odours.
- Dysosmia: distorted odor perceptions in the presence of an odor source (parosmia) or odor perception in the absence of a stimulant odor (phantosmia).
- Cacosmia: a normally pleasant odour is detected as foul or unpleasant.
- Heterosmia: the inability to smell one of the few odours in the presence of an otherwise-normal sense of smell.

- Agnosia: inability to contrast or classify odours, although with the ability to detect them.
    (1) Conduction, (2) Sensorial, or (3) Neural smell loss

Etiologies of Olfactory Dysfunction

- Sinonasal diseases
    - Upper respiratory tract infections (especially viral)
    - Allergic rhinitis
    - Non-allergic rhinitis (medicamentosa, vasomotora, atrophic)
    - Chronic rhinosinusitis
    - Nasal polyps
    - Adenoid hypertrophy
    - Benign tumour
    - Malignant tumour
- Trauma
    - Head trauma (damage to cribriform plate)
    - Postsurgical skull base
    - Post-lobotomy (frontal, temporal)
    - Ensocopic surgery
- Neurodegenerative diseases
    - Alzheimer's disease
    - Parkinson disease
    - Multiple sclerosis
- Endocrine–metabolic disorders
    - Diabetes mellitus
    - Hypothyroidism
    - Pregnancy
    - Adrenal cortical insufficiency
    - Cushing's syndrome
    - Chronic renal failure
    - Cirrhosis of the liver
- Nutritional deficiencies
    - Vitamin deficiency (A, B6, B12)
    - Zinc deficiency
- Neurologic diseases
    - CNS tumour
    - AVM
    - Multiple sclerosis
    - Epilepsy

- Medications
  - Chemotherapeutic agents
  - Amitriptyline hydrochloride
  - Nifedipine
  - Propranolol hydrochloride
  - Labetalol hydrochloride
  - Radioactive iodine
- Miscellaneous
  - Kallman's syndrome
  - Post-radiation
  - Total laryngectomy
  - Postanaesthesia
  - Schizophrenia
  - Down's and Turner's syndromes
  - Alcoholism
  - Toxic chemical exposure (Ammonia, hairdressing chemicals, gasoline, formaldehyde, paint solvents)

Diagnosis

- History
- Physical examination
- Laboratory tests
- CT of the sinuses and nose: highly diagnostic for sinonasal pathology
- MRI of brain: in patients with suspicion of intracranial lesions
- Olfactory testing: University of Pennsylvania smell identification test

Therapy

<u>Therapy of the underlying cause</u>.

- Endocrine disturbances should be addressed
- Nutritional deficiencies should be corrected.
- Some drugs should be discontinued.
- The use of oral and/or intranasal steroids may be useful.
- Patients with chronic rhinosinusitis and/or polyps can benefit from endoscopic sinus surgery.

2.32   Fibrous Dysplasia

Developmental anomaly characterized by replacement of normal bone with proliferating fibrous tissue and immature woven bone.

– More common in maxilla during the first two decades.

Forms

– Monostotic form: in a single bone (70%)
– Polyostotic form: in multiple bones

Diagnosis

– Radiological examination: radiolucent areas which later develop into a partially opaque ground glass appearance.
– Difficult distinction between fibrous dysplasia and ossifying fibromas (capsule formation)

Therapy

Surgical (in patients with progressive symptoms or when the disease threatens important anatomical structures)

– Radical excision of all dysplastic bone (this procedure may cause further deformities).
– Some reports indicate that surgery may activate the tumor and accelerate the growth.

2.33   Pyogenic Granuloma (Lobular Capillary Hemangioma)

A rapidly growing benign capillary hemangioma of unknown aetiology.

– The term "pyogenic granuloma" is a misnomer (the disease it is neither infectious nor granulomatous).

- It most commonly occurs in women in the second and third decade of life, which is likely related to the high incidence of pregnancy during this time period.
- It affects the skin and mucosal lining of the oral cavity and nose (anterior septum is the most frequently affected followed by turbinate).

Predisposing factors

1. Hormonal stimulation during pregnancy
2. Trauma to mucosa (habitual nasal picking, prolonged contact with irritating agents from nasal packing, nasogastric tube, foreign body or nose piercing)
3. Oral contraceptives.

Symptoms

- Unilateral recurrent epistaxis
- Nasal obstruction

Diagnosis

- Nasal endoscopy: raised or polypoidal mass with surface ulceration, which may or may not be present.

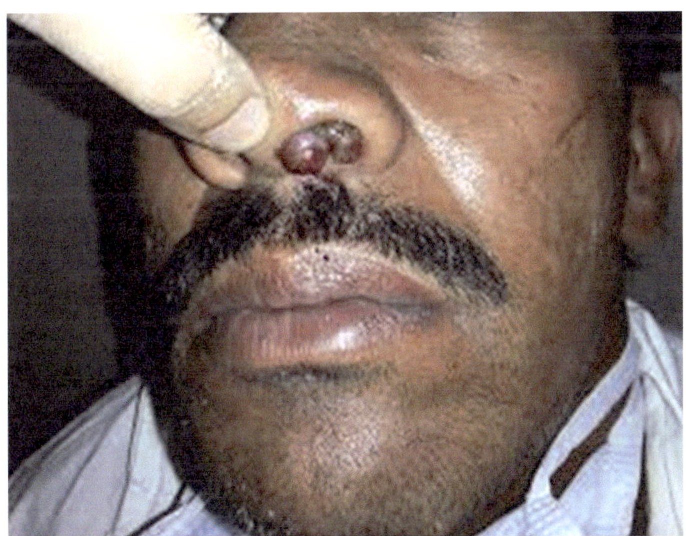

- CT scan: non-specific features of a well-defined soft tissue density mass with a hypoattenuating cap of variable thickness.

Therapy
Conservative

- Observation: spontaneous resolution is frequent after pregnancy ends

Surgical

- Endoscopic surgical resection and cauterization: in patients who experience severe bouts of epistaxis or whose lesions fail to resolve after pregnancy.

2.34   Squamous Papilloma

Squamous papillomas (SPs) are common benign lesions occurring in the entirety of the upper aerodigestive tract.

- Low risk of recurrence and malignant transformation.
- Associated with HPV serotypes 6 and 11.
- Most common sites: nasal vestibule and caudal septum

Symptoms

- Nasal obstruction

Diagnosis

- Nasal endoscopy: Gross appearance varies from pale to fleshy pink, and they may be sessile or pedunculated.

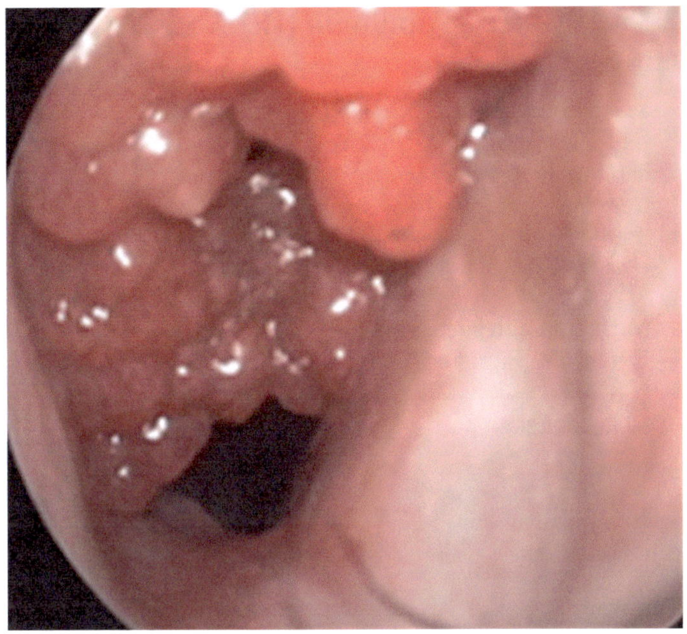

Therapy

– Removal of the SP is generally recommended in order to relieve symptoms and to exclude the possibility of malignancy.

Surgical

– Surgical resection may be accomplished endoscopically or by direct visualization of lesions in the nasal vestibule.

Conservative

– In selected patients careful observation is an acceptable.

2.35   Inverted Papilloma (IP)

A locally aggressive, benign nasal lesion remarkable for its tendency for local recurrence and association with carcinoma. It is characterized by proliferation of epithelium into the underlying stroma.

– Most common site of origin: lateral nasal wall.
– Extension into: maxillary sinus (69%), sphenoid sinus (11–20%)
– **10% change to SCC**

Symptoms

– Nasal obstruction
– Rhinorrhea
– Epistaxis
– Headache
– Facial pressure

Diagnosis

– Nasal endoscopy: it is firmer and less translucent than a nasal polyp.
– CT scan: Bone destruction due to pressure from the tumor
– Biopsy: the proliferated epithelium is found to be invaginated towards stroma.

Therapy

Wide excision with normal surrounding tissue is necessary to prevent recurrence.

– Endoscopically
– Transnasally
– Lateral rhinotomy approach
– Midfacial degloving

COMPLICATION
High recurrence rate

2.36   Juvenile Naso-Pharyngeal Angiofibroma

A rare, benign, highly vascular tumour of predominantly adolescent males that originates in postero-lateral nasal cavity, around SPF.

– Vascular supply: most common internal maxillary art.
– It may locally behave aggressively.

It can extend:

Anteriorly: nasal cavity
Superiorly: sphenoid sinus
Posteriorly: nasopharynx
Laterally: pterygo-palantine fossa, infratemporal fossa.

Symptoms

– Nasal obstruction
– Epistaxis
– Headache
– Eustachean tube obstruction
– Nasal speech

Symptoms indicating advanced disease

– Ocular symptoms
– Cranial nerve palsies

Diagnosis

1. Endoscopy
2. CT:
   • Homogeneously enhancing mass in the posterior nasal cavity and nasopharynx
   • Widening of pterygo-palantine fossa
   • Anterior bowing of posterior maxillary wall (Hollman-Miller sign).

3. MRI: intermediate signal on T1 images, high signal on T2 images.
4. External carotid arteriogram
5. **Biopsy can be dangerous!**

Therapy

Preoperative embolization (minimizes blood loss) + Surgical resection

Surgical approaches: The surgical approach should be selected according to the location and the extent of the tumour, the tumour vasculature, the effectiveness of the embolization, the age of the patient, and the experience of the surgical team

1. Open surgery: transpalatal approach, lateral rhinotomy, midfacial degloving (popular, because it avoids any facial scars), craniofacial approach (intracranial extension).
2. Combined open and endoscopic surgery: to allow close inspection of the surgical cavity and to allow for further resection, if necessary
3. Endoscopic surgery alone: has limitations and is not suitable for tumours with extensive intra-cranial extension, extension lateral to the cavernous sinus, or posterior to the pterygoid plates

2.37   Malignant Tumours

Sites of predilection

- Maxillary s 60–70%
- Nasal cavity 20–30%
- Ethmoid s 10–15%
- Frontal/sphenoid ‹5%

Types

- Squamous cell carcinoma 60–70%
- Adenocarcinoma 10–20%
- Rhabdomyosarcoma (in children)
- ENB
- ACC
- Melanoma
- Undifferentiated

<u>Risk factors</u>
- Wood dust
- Nickel
- Leather
- Textile dust
- Asbestos
  - **Ohngren** divided the sinus into halves by an imaginary plane passing through the medial canthus of the eye and the angle of the mandible.
- Infrastructure tumours: present earlier, are more amenable to resection and have better prognosis.
- Suprastructure lesions: present later, are challenging to resect due to proximity to pterygopalatine fossa, infratemporal fossa, orbit and skull base.

Symptoms

- Nasal obstruction
- Hyposmia
- Epistaxis
- Feeling of pressure or headache.

If they occur unilaterally this might be the first indication of a tumour.

<u>Signs of extensive tumour</u>

- Visual disturbance (e.g. reduction of vision, double vision),
- CSF leak, meningitis,
- External swelling of the cheek or forehead,
- Epiphora
- Irritation of the first or second branch of the trigeminal nerve (hyper-esthesia and pain).

Diagnosis

1. Inspection: assessment of facial asymmetry
2. Palpation of the neck: assessment for LN spread.
3. Intraoral examination: check the integrity of the palate and upper gingiva.
4. Mandibular excursion should be assessed for trismus (signifies expansion into the pterygoid space).

5. Otoscopy: for effusion related to Eustachian tube dysfunction.
6. Visual acuity, pupillary response, extra-ocular motion
7. Cranial nerve deficits
8. CT and MRI: evaluation of location and extent of the lesion, surgical planning and post-operative follow-up.
9. The vascularisation of lesion can be evaluated with digital subtraction angiography.
10. If tumor involves ICA, a balloon occlusion test should be performed along with a perfusion scintigraphy of the brain. It gives information as to if the ICA can be sacrificed.
11. In cases with suspected CSF leak a CT or MR cisternography might be helpful.

Therapy

<u>Surgical removal and post-operative radiotherapy</u>

- Inoperable cases: adjuvant chemoradiotherapy.
- T1 & T2: Endonasal micro-endoscopic tumor surgery.
- T3 & T4: classical external approaches (lateral rhinotomy, midfacial degloving, anterior craniofacial resection)

<u>Surgical principles</u>

- Intraoperatively frozen sections should be obtained to ensure complete tumor removal.
- Periorbital infiltration → periorbit removed and reconstructed
- Dura removal → duraplasty
- A criticism of endonasal approach is the impossibility to obtain en bloc resection. It is accepted, however, to resect larger tumors segmentally.
- *Orbit*: Involved periorbit can be resected with preservation of orbital contents when there is no invasion of (1) orbital fat, (2) muscles or (3) orbital apex. Invasion of any of these structures is an indication for orbital exenteration.
- *Neck*: In cases of resectable primary tumors with clinically and radiologically N+ should be managed with some form of ND.

The management of N0s debatable: the way of lymphatic spread can be to the prevertebral and retropharyngeal nodes as well as to the cervical nodes, and classical ND may therefore leave residual disease. Thus, elective ND is not advised in sinonasal malignancy (thus, thorough neck investigations are mandatory during patient follow-up).

Advantages of endonasal approach:

- Optimal overview over the entire paranasal sinus system.
- Dura defects can be reliably closed exclusively endonasally.
- The bony boundaries of the surgical field can be preserved → less danger for cele formation and reduced disturbance for the growing midfacial skeleton in children.
- Avoid visible scars.

Limitations to the use of microendoscopic approach:

- Extensive involvement of the frontal sinus
- Extensive intracranial infiltration
- Intraorbital infiltration
- If a tumour originates from the posterolateral, anterior or inferior wall of the maxillary sinus
- Recurrent lesions associated with massive scar tissue
- **Follow-up**: Endoscopy and MRI
    - Clinical controls quarterly in the 1st& 2nd year, semi-annually in 3rd year and thereafter only annually.
    - MRI of paranasal sinuses, skull base and neck (to exclude LN metastases): 3 months after surgery. Afterwards yearly.
    - CT: yearly, since solitary metastases are resectable.
    - Prognosis (from favourable to poor): ENB, ACC, ADC, SCC, melanoma, undifferentiated

Esthesioneuroblastoma

- Kadish staging system: extent of disease

Squamous cell carcinoma

- Risk factors: nickel, mustard gas, chromium

Adenoid Cystic carcinoma

- Perineural spread

Adenocarcinoma

- Associated with exposure to wood dust, lacquers

Melanomas

- They account for less than 1% of all melanomas
- Ballantyne's clinical staging system

Rhabdomyosarcoma

- Frequently found in children

Further Readings

1. Ponikau JU, Sherris DA, Kern EB, Homburger HA, Frigas E, Gaffey TA, Roberts GD. The diagnosis and incidence of allergic fungal sinusitis. Mayo Clin Proc. 1999;74(9):877–84.
2. Orlandi RR, Kingdom TT, Hwang PH, Smith TL, Alt JA, Baroody FM, Batra PS, Bernal-Sprekelsen M, et al. International consensus statement on allergy and rhinology: rhinosinusitis. Int Forum Allergy Rhinol. 2016;6(Suppl 1):S22–209.
3. Ensenat J, de Notaris M, Sanchez M, Fernandez C, Ferrer E, Bernal-Sprekelsen M, Alobid I. Endoscopic endonasal surgery for skull base tumours: technique and preliminary results in a consecutive case series report. Rhinology. 2013;51(1):37–46.
4. Fokkens WJ, Lund VJ, Mullol J, Bachert C, Alobid I, Baroody F, Cohen N, Cervin A, Douglas R, Gevaert P, Georgalas C, Goossens H, Harvey R, Hellings P, Hopkins C, Jones N, Joos G, Kalogjera L, Kern B, Kowalski M, Price D, Riechelmann H, Schlosser R, Senior B, Thomas M, Toskala E, Voegels R, Wang de Y, Wormald PJ. European position paper on rhinosinusitis and nasal polyps. Rhinol Suppl. 2012;23:3. preceding table of contents, 1–298.
5. Greiner AN, Hellings PW, Rotiroti G, Scadding GK. Allergic rhinitis. Lancet. 2011;378(9809):2112–22.
6. Wojciechowska J, Krajewski W, Krajewski P, Kręcicki T. Granulomatosis with polyangiitis in otolaryngologist practice:

a review of current knowledge. Clin Exp Otorhinolaryngol. 2016;9(1):8–13.

 7. Zuniga MG, Turner JH. Treatment outcomes in acute invasive fungal rhinosinusitis. Curr Opin Otolaryngol Head Neck Surg. 2014;22(3):242–8.

 8. Kim YS, Kim K, Lee JG, Yoon JH, Kim CH. Paranasal sinus mucoceles with ophthalmologic manifestations: a 17-year review of 96 cases. Am J Rhinol Allergy. 2011;25(4):272–5.

 9. Kochhar A, Byrne PJ. Surgical management of complex midfacial fractures. Otolaryngol Clin N Am. 2013;46(5):759–78.

10. Khoueir N, Nicolas N, Rohayem Z, Haddad A, Abou Hamad W. Exclusive endoscopic resection of juvenile nasopharyngeal angiofibroma: a systematic review of the literature. Otolaryngol Head Neck Surg. 2014;150(3):350–8.

11. Wood JW, Casiano RR. Inverted papillomas and benign non-neoplastic lesions of the nasal cavity. Am J Rhinol Allergy. 2012;26(2):157–63.

Chapter 3
Larynx

3.1 Laryngomalacia

> Supraglottis is flaccid and epiglottis or inter-arytenoid tissue collapse during inspiration to obstruct the airway.

– The most common cause of neonatal stridor.

<u>Classification.</u>

type 1: tight or fore-shortened aryepiglottic folds.
type 2: redundant tissue.
type 3: epiglottic collapse due to underlying neuromuscular disorders.

Symptoms

– Stridor (soon after birth): worse with crying and lying in the supine position

Diagnosis

– Flexible endoscopy: "omega" shaped epiglottis that falls backward during inspiration.
– Operative endoscopy: if stridor is very severe with cyanosis.

P. Koltsidopoulos et al., *ENT*,
DOI 10.1007/978-3-319-56330-5_3,

Therapy

- Observation and assurance that it will resolve by 12–16 months.
- Endoscopic epiglottoplasty for severe stridor.
- Tracheotomy may be required.

3.2   Neonatal Laryngeal Paralysis

The second most common cause of neonatal stridor.

Causes:

- Idiopathic
- Birth trauma
- History of cardiac surgery
- Neurologic disease: Arnold-Chiari malformation
- Malignant disease (brainstem lesions)

Symptoms

- Weak cry
- Inspiratory stridor
- Feeding difficulties

Diagnosis

- Fiberoptic endoscopy
- Imaging: to rule out cardiac and neurologic causes.
- Barium swallow: advisable to detect aspiration.

Therapy

- Observation (for mild stridor)
- Tracheotomy (for severe stridor)
- Definitive laryngeal surgery deferred pending potential recovery and growth.
- Laryngeal reinnervation reported effective, usually around age 5.

3.3   Laryngeal Hemangioma

Vascular lesion that causes airway obstruction.

Symptoms

– Progressive inspiratory stridor (onset soon after birth).
– Progressive episodes of croup.
– Voice usually normal.
– Skin hemangioma (in 50% of cases).

Diagnosis

– Direct laryngoscopy and bronchoscopy: compressible, erythematous lesion most often involving the anterior
  subglottis.
– Imaging: to assess the extent.
  • Do not biopsy

Therapy

– Observation (natural history is expansion followed by
  involution).
– Systemic steroids and epinephrine for stridor.
– Systemic propranolol
– CO_2 laser excision, external excision or tracheotomy if
  obstruction does not respond to propranolol.

3.4   Laryngeal Web or Atresia

A congenital band over part (web) or all (atresia) of the
glottis.

– Webs usually involve anterior larynx.

Symptoms

- Small web: asymptomatic.
- Large web: weak or hoarse cry.
- Laryngeal atresia presents with complete obstruction at birth, unless a distal T-E fistula exists.

Diagnosis

- Endoscopic examination

Therapy

- Tracheotomy for relief
- Web is best corrected when child is larger and anatomy is more distinct.

3.5   Subglottic Stenosis

Narrowing of the subglottic airway, which is housed in the cricoid cartilage.

Etiology

- Congenital
- Acquired: trauma/intubation, chronic infection, chronic inflammatory disease, neoplastic disease

Cotton–Myer grading system

  I. <50%
 II. 51–70%
III. 71–99%
IV. no detectable lumen, complete obliteration

Therapy
Surgical treatment

- Grade I/II: laser, dilation, cold knife
- Grade III/IV: tracheostomy, laryngotracheal reconstruction (cricoid split with anterior ± posterior cricoid augmentation), cricotracheal resection

- Single stage (no postoperative tracheotomy present) versus double stage (persistent postoperative tracheotomy with staged decannulation)

3.6   Acute Laryngitis

Inflammation of the larynx.

<u>Etiology</u>

- URI: laryngeal inflammation usually results from coughing, not direct infection.
- Voice abuse: shouting and loud talking require tight closure
- Gastroesophageal reflux
- Any combination of the above

Symptoms

- Interarytenoid edema limits glottis closure. Voice may be rough, weak or breathy and increased adductor effort is required to speak.
- Hoarseness
- No dyspnea

Diagnosis

- History
    - Sudden onset of hoarseness
    - Inciting factor (URI, voice abuse, reflux)
    - Reflux should be suspected if hoarseness occurs after a patient has gone to bed soon after a large meal.
- Routine head and neck examination: seeks signs of URI, sinusitis.
- Laryngeal examination: to rule out other causes of hoarseness.
    (a) assure normal vocal fold motion
    (b) no lesions on VF
    (c) look for interarytenoid edema.

Therapy
Vocal hygiene (absolute silence not required)

1. Hydration
2. Mucolytic
3. Decongestants for nasal obstruction
4. Cough suppression
5. H2 blockers or proton pump inhibitors (if acid reflux is detected)
6. Steroids only for urgent need to use voice.
   - Avoid drying antihistamines
   - Natural History: it resolves spontaneously over 1–2 weeks.
   - Laryngitis precipitated by one factor may be prolonged by other factors (GORD, voice abuse)

3.7   Candidiasis

Risk factors: Inhaled steroids, antibiotic therapy, immune compromise, acid reflux.

Diagnosis

- History: progressive hoarseness, cough and globus sensation.
- Laryngoscopy: white patches on bright red mucosa.

   D/D: leukoplakia.

Therapy

- Systemic antifungal treatment.
- Withhold steroid.

3.8   Epiglottitis

Infection of supraglottis.

Causative agent: **Haemophilus influenza**

- It primarily affects children (3–6 years) and follows a bout of rhinopharyngitis.
- If untreated, death can occur within a few hours.

Symptoms

- Sore throat
- Dysphagia
- "Hot potato" voice
- Drooling (mouth falls open to allow the saliva that is too difficult to swallow to dribble out.)
- Fever
- Dyspnea (relieved somewhat by leaning forward)
- Stridor

Diagnosis

- History
- Point tenderness at the hyoid level in midline.
- Flexible endoscopy
- (<u>Examination should be gentle to avoid stimulating a gag, which can precipitate sudden upper airway obstruction</u>. Do not use a tongue blade)
- Imaging should not delay treatment.
- In doubtful cases a lateral soft tissue shows the swollen epiglottis.
- A CT may demonstrate the rare occurrence of an abscess of epiglottis.
- Any patient sent for imaging for suspected epiglottitis should be continuously attended by a physician capable of emergency airway management.
- Blood cultures are more likely than mucosal cultures to document the pathogen.

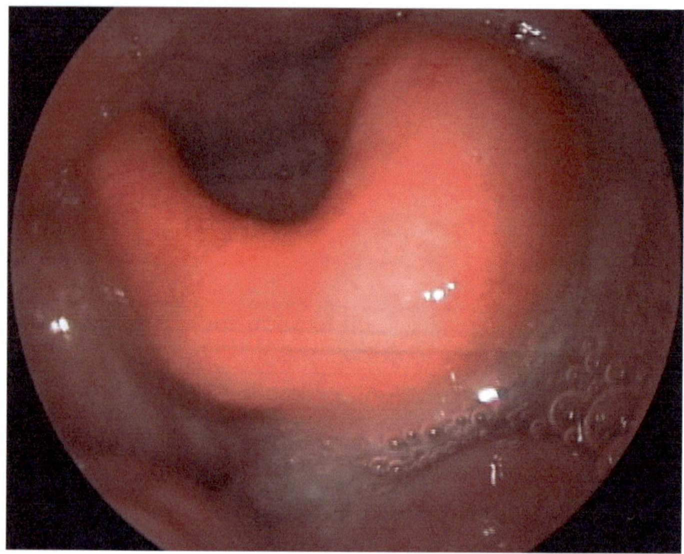

Therapy

– <u>Establish airway with tracheotomy or intubation.</u>
– (Selected adults without severe stridor may be managed only with close monitoring.)
– Intravenous antibiotics effective against H. influenzae [such ascefotaxime (Claforan), 200 mg/kg per day].
– Steroids. They are of little effect on their own.

3.9   Croup Acute

Infection of the upper airway, which obstructs breathing and causes a characteristic barking cough.

– Primarily in children between 1 and 3 years.

Causative agents: parainfluenza types 1–4, H. influenza, streptococci, staphylococci or pneumococci.

Symptoms

- Barking cough
- Hoarseness
- Inspiratory stridor
- Respiratory distress

Diagnosis

- History
- Physical examination: supra-sternal retractions and accessory muscle use, agitation and increased pulse (signs of hypercarbia), circumoral pallor and cyanosis (late signs).
- Imaging: "steeple" sign on soft tissue anteroposterior image (subglottic narrowing due to edema).

  D/D: epiglottitis, and inhalation of a foreign body.

Therapy

- Cool mist inhalation
- Steroids
- Humidified oxygen, intermittent racemic epinephrine.
- Antibiotics (if indicated by fever or culture)
- Airway intervention (if obstruction is severe)
- Recurrent croup is an indication for operative endoscopy, due to possible subglottic stenosis.

3.10   Vocal Nodules

> Chronic thickenings of VC epithelium, usually located at the junction of the anterior third with the middle third.

Groups prone to vocal nodules: women, male children, people with occupations with highly demanding vocal activity (teachers, singers, salesman, etc.).

Etiological factors: vocal abuse, occasionally severe coughing.

Diagnosis

- History
- Laryngoscopy: opposing, usually symmetric masses of the middle portion of the membranous vocal fold.

Therapy

- Voice restriction or rest
- Voice therapy
- Occasionally surgical removal

3.11   Vocal Fold Polyp

Benign lesions usually located at the vocal edge of the VC, impeding VCs meeting while adducting.

- Mainly in adult males.
  Risk factors: vocal abuse, anxiety and extroverted behaviour, noisy environment at work, excessive sphincteric function of the larynx (weight lifting, glass-blowing, etc.).
  Pathophysiology: Result of a violent and short voice strength that leads to rupture of capillaries in the submucosa, with subsequent haemorrhage. If voice misuse continues, the initial lesion can evolve to a haemorrhagic polyp or, after some time, to a fibrotic polyp.

Symptoms

- Hoarseness
- Bleeding into polyp can cause sudden enlargement.
- Dysphonia is usually abrupt, coincident with the vocal abuse. Later on, dysphonia can be intermittent or continuous, depending on the polyp structure and localization.
- Vocal range is reduced and conversational voice appears muffled, with difficulty to achieve high-pitched tones.
- Polyps can become large, producing even glottis obstruction.

Diagnosis

- History: chronic hoarseness, recurring bouts of laryngitis.
- Indirect laryngoscopy:
  - Smooth soft tissue mass, usually pale
  - Usually unilateral
  - Located in the membranous portion of the vocal cord.
  - They have either a wide or a narrow pedicle
  - They may have a contact lesion in the contra-lateral VC.
  - Large polyps move up and down in the glottis along with the respiratory movements.

Therapy

- Excision via direct microlaryngoscopy.
  - Microsurgical technique is directed to polyp removal by cutting its pedicle and avoiding disrupting the vocal ligament.
  - Endoscopic laser removal has also been proposed.
- Medical treatment is not important in polyp treatment, other than changing or removing the possible harmful medications (aspirin, warfarin).
  - If gastropharyngeal reflux is present, adequate antireflux measures should be applied.
  - Although speech therapy is not essential, postsurgical rehabilitation is recommended to teach the patient good vocal hygiene habits.

3.12   Reinke's Edema

A unilateral or bilateral swelling of the vocal cord characterized by the accumulation of gelatinlike material in Reinke's space.

Pathophysiology: chronic irritation of the larynx leads to accumulation of fluid, a consequence of poor lymphatic drainage, vascular congestion and venous stasis.

<u>Etiology</u>

- Smoking
- Voice misuse
- Long history of dysphonia

Other possible causes

- Chronic sinusitis
- Hypothyroidism
- Exposure to industrial or environmental irritants

Symptoms

- Vocal pitch is low, with females having a male tone.
- Speech parameters include a narrow vocal range as well as a reduction in the fundamental frequency.
- Occasionally, the oedema may be big enough to reduce the glottic space, causing dyspnoea.

Diagnosis

- Laryngoscopy: Fusiform oedema in both vocal cords. Sometimes a yellow fluid content can be seen through the vocal cord mucosa.
- Stroboscopy: shows a complete glottis closure, with asymmetric movement of the vocal cords, and an overexpressed mucosal wave, whose stiffness is severely reduced.

Therapy
Conservative treatment

- Initial measures are directed to avoid irritants and follow speech therapy.

  Voice improvement takes time, and should be monitored periodically by indirect laryngoscopy.

Surgical treatment

– In advanced cases, or when conservative measures do not improve the voice.
– Cordotomy in the superior aspect of the vocal cord, and aspiration of the fluid present in Reinke's space.
– Redundant mucosa is removed with microscissors.
– Stripping should be avoided owing to the multiple micro-adherences between the mucosa.

3.13   Vocal Cord Cysts

Benign masses of the membranous vocal folds.

Symptoms

– The symptoms are similar to those produced by nodules.
– Vocal misuse is a frequent clinical characteristic, with dysphonia as the most constant clinical symptom.
– Spontaneous opening of the cyst produces a sudden improvement of voice quality
– Spontaneous rupture of the cyst is thought to be the origin of sulcus vocalis.

Diagnosis

• History: A long-lasting history of dysphonia and vocal abuse.
• Laryngoscopy shows a white, soft, smooth, fusiform elevation of the middle third of the VC, sometimes with a contra lateral VC contact lesion.
• Epidermoid cysts are larger, ovoid, yellow and sometimes bilateral, with greater effect on voice quality than retention cysts, which tend to be smaller, white and unilateral.
• Stroboscopy: increase of fundamental frequency with the characteristic stop of the mucosal wave in the cyst area, maintaining a normal wave progression in the mucosa anterior and posterior to the cyst.

Therapy

- Surgery is the treatment of choice: Superior cordotomy and cyst detachment from the underlying mucosa.
- Corticoid injections in the vocalis muscle have also been recommended to avoid postoperative inflammation and adherence between the epithelium and the vocal ligament.
- Speech therapy is indicated to improve voice habits in the postoperative period.

3.14 Laryngocele

Dilation of laryngeal ventricle, filled with air or fluid.

1. *Internal*: within thyroid cartilage framework.
2. *External*: herniates through thryrohyoid membrane.
3. *Combined*

<u>Risk factors</u>

1. excessive cough
2. playing wind instruments, glassblowers 3. obstructing lesion, e.g. tumour

Finding of a laryngocele should prompt a search for an underlying laryngeal carcinoma.

Symptoms

- Hoarseness
- Swelling in the neck that may increase in size with "Valsava" maneuver (external laryngocele).

Diagnosis

- Indirect laryngoscopy: enlargement of the false vocal fold or entire supraglottis.

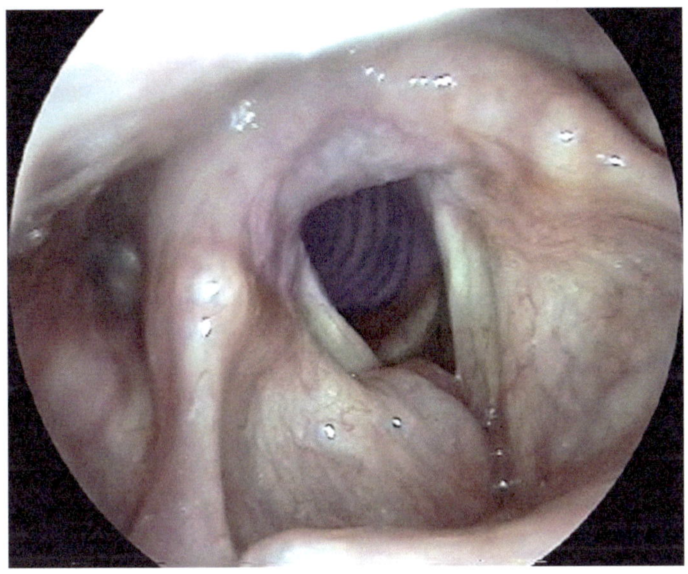

- CT: a well defined, air or fluid filled lesion related to the paraglottic space, which has continuity with the laryngeal ventricle.

Therapy

- Internal: endoscopic marsupialization
- External or recurrent: external approach.

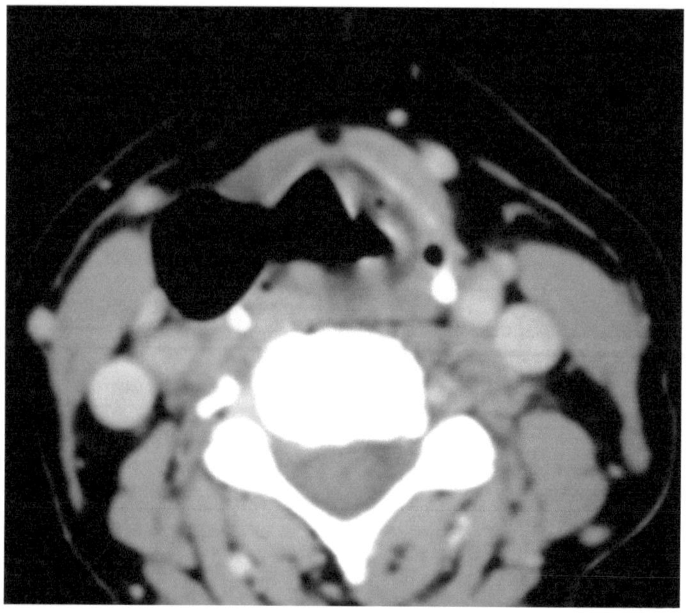

3.15 Laryngeal Papillomatosis

Benign warty tumor caused by human papilloma virus (types 6 and 11).

- Primary site of involvement is larynx.
- Other sites: trachea, bronchi, pharynx, tonsils.
- Maternal transmission from mothers with genital warts.

Symptoms

- Hoarseness (early sign)
- Stridor and shortness of breath (later signs)

Diagnosis

- Indirect laryngoscopy
- Direct laryngoscopy and biopsy for definitive diagnosis.

Therapy

- Micro-laryngoscopy and excision: microdebrider, CO_2 laser, or microsurgical instruments.
  Office based endoscopic procedures with local anesthesia can be used in some adults.
  Other treatments: cryotherapy, photodynamic therapy, injection of anti-virals (cidofovir)
- Frequent recurrence of the disease.
- Malignant transformation may occur (subtypes 16 and 18)
- Tracheotomy should be avoided as lesions may spread and implant further down in the airway.

3.16   Laryngeal Chondroma

A rare, benign, slowly growing tumor of the larynx.

Sites: posterior plate of the cricoid cartilage (the most frequent), thyroid, arytenoids, and epiglottis.

Symptoms

- Hoarseness
- Dyspnea
- Dysphagia
- Globus sensation.

Diagnosis

- Indirect laryngoscopy: submucosal mass
- CT scanning (the lesion is often only apparent on CT scanning).
  - Differential diagnosis between chondromas and chondrosarcomas can be difficult.

Therapy

Surgical excision

A. thyrotomy for anterior tumors.
B. lateral approach for other areas.
   - Recurrence is common

3.17 Hyperplastic Epithelial Lesions

A hyperplastic and dysplastic stage (keratinization) of epithelial lesions in the glottic region that may or may not develop into an invasive carcinoma.

<u>Classification of premalignant laryngeal lesions.</u>
Keratosis and leukoplakia are premalignant epithelial lesions of laryngeal mucosa.
Etiology: smoking, vocal abuse, chronic laryngitis, GERD and vitamin deficiencies.

Symptoms

– Hoarseness

Diagnosis

- Laryngoscopy: thickened white or reddish patches.
- Stroboscopy: lesions usually impair glottal closure, but restriction of mucosal wave suggests invasive cancer.
- Biopsy

Therapy

A. Conservative: cessation of smoking, antireflux therapy and voice therapy.
B. Direct laryngoscopy with excisional biopsy.
C. Periodic follow-up to detect recurrence.

3.18 Spasmodic Dysphonia (SD)

Intermittent involuntary spasms of intrinsic laryngeal muscles during speech.

Unknown etiology

A. ADductor form
   - most frequent
   - strained and strangled voice with frequent voice breaks.
B. ABductor form
   - 1 in 10 patients with SD.
   - whispering or breathy voice

Laryngeal muscles	
Adductor	Lateral cricoarytenoid
Abductor	Posterior cricoarytenoid
Tensor	Cricothyroid

Diagnosis

A. Based on perceptual assessment and laryngeal examination to rule out anatomic pathology.
B. Diagnostic criteria
   - patient perceives increased effort in speaking.
   - difficulty fluctuates over time and between tasks.
   - symptoms have lasted more than 3 months
   - one or more of these vocal tasks are normal: laugh, cry, shout, whisper, sing or yawn.
   - normal laryngeal anatomy and normal function for non-speech tasks

Therapy

- Speech therapy alone has very limited efficacy.
- RLN transection (symptoms often recur within 3 years).
- Botulinum toxin injection of the thyro-arytenoid muscle (the most widely used treatment for AD-SD)
- Botulinum toxin injection into the posterior cricoarytenoid muscle (for AB-SD).

- Surgical treatment
  - "Berke procedure" (transects adductor branches of RLN and reinnervates with branches of ansa cervicalis).
  - Medialization thyroplasty (AB-SD)
  - Lateralization thyroplasty (AD-SD).

3.19   Rheumatoid Arthritis

Rheumatoid arthritis can cause inflammatory fixation of the cricoarytenoid joint and inflammatory nodules on the vocal fold.

Symptoms

- Hoarseness
- Pain
- Globus
- Referred otalgia
- Bilateral arthritis causes dyspnea and stridor.

Diagnosis

- History of rheumatoid arthritis.
- Laryngoscopy: immobile arytenoid with erythema and edema in arthritis.
- Serology: elevated ESR, RF, decreased complement levels
- HR CT: can show erosion of joint and soft tissue lesion.

Therapy

- Steroids
- Tracheotomy may be required to relieve airway obstruction.

3.20   Relapsing Polychondritis

Uncommon chronic inflammatory disease involving cartilaginous structures, predominantly those of the ears, nose, and laryngotracheobronchial tree.

Symptoms

- Commonly begins with painful swelling and erythema of auricles.
- Stridor (due to progressive cartilage destruction-50%)

Diagnosis

- History
- Physical examination
- Biopsy is nonspecific, but may exclude other etiologies.

Therapy

- Initially high dose steroids
- Maintenance with low-dose steroids and methtrexate.
- Airway protection (possible tracheotomy)
- Airway disease can progress to death from pneumonia or obstructive respiratory failure.

3.21   Amyloidosis

Clinical disorder characterized by accumulation of amyloid (an abnormal fibrillar protein) within tissues and organs causing alteration of their normal function.

- It can attack any organ.
- It frequently affects the heart, kidneys, liver, spleen, nervous system and digestive tract.
- It can lead to life-threatening organ failure.
- Primary, secondary or myeloma-associated.

Symptoms

- Hoarseness
- Dyspnea, stridor
- Dysphagia
- Globus
- Enlarged tongue

Diagnosis

- Laryngoscopy: waxy lesions that may be gray or orange typically on the epiglottis, but sometimes glottis or subglottic.

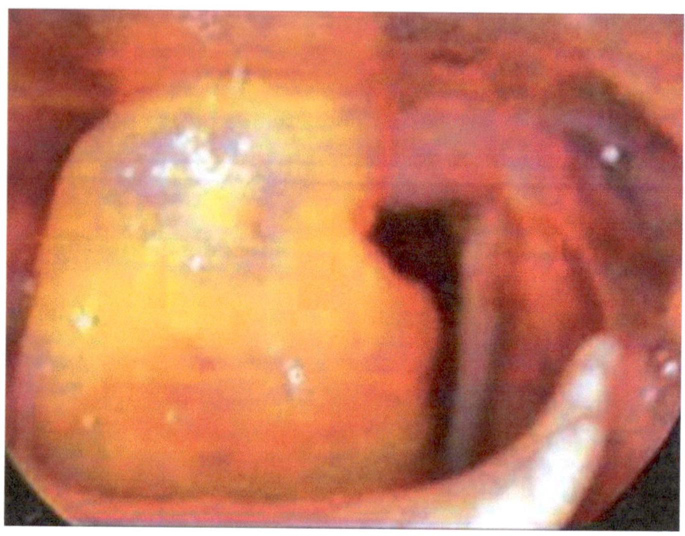

- Biopsy: apple green birefringence with Congo red staining viewed under polarizing light.

Therapy

- Endoscopic excision or open surgery to remove or debulk symptomatic lesions.
  - Total removal is often impossible.
  - Frequent recurrence.

3.22   Laryngeal Cancer

<u>Types</u>
- SCC: the commonest (95%)
- Other primary malignant tumors: salivary gland tumors, neurological tumors and chondromas.

- Secondary: laryngeal metastases from other malignant tumours (melanoma, hypernephroma) or laryngeal manifestations of general or systemic malignancies (non-Hodgkin's lymphoma).

Risk factors: smoking, alcohol, HPV, history of prior head and neck SCC.

Premalignant laryngeal lesions: spectrum from hyperplasia, atypia, dysplasia (mild/moderate/severe), carcinoma in situ (CIS).

Symptoms

Supraglottic:
- Odynophagia, referred otalgia, dysphagia, globus sensation.
- Most common subsite involved is the epiglottis.
- Spread to base of tongue or pre-epiglottic space.
- 25–50% have nodal metastases to cervical LN at the time of presentation.
  (spreads to levels II–IV, increased risk of contralateral neck)

Glottic carcinoma:
- hoarseness, globus.
- most common site of laryngeal cancer
- low incidence of cervical metastasis.
- tumors extend through ventricle, anterior commissure, and paraglottic space.

Subglottic:
- airway obstruction, dyspnea, stridor, progressive dysphagia
- rare and aggressive

Diagnosis

- History of a sore throat, dysphonia, dysphagia, otalgia and/ or a neck mass.
- Indirect laryngoscopy:
  Site and size of the tumour, mobility of VCs
  Tumors located in the ventricle, the epiglottis, and the sub-glottis may escape detection.

- Palpation of the neck: to detect adenopathy. Frequent at the time of diagnosis, more so with supraglottic than with glottic cancers. These palpable or involved LN are most often located in the subdigastric (level IIa) and midjugular (level III) nodal levels.

  The size, site and mobility of all nodes should be documented.

  Examination of the neck may also reveal signs of direct extension of the cancer into the tissues of the neck.

  Pain generated by the movement of the thyroid cartilage is suggestive of an extension into the neck.

- CT from the nasopharynx to the upper mediastinum: to assess the location and size of the primary cancer and to evaluate extension to the neck.

  A cancer of the vocal cord or the ventricle may extend into the paraglottic space, and supraglottic cancer can extend to invade the pre-epiglottic space.

  The probability of metastatic involvement of LNs is associated with the following criteria seen on imaging:

  → Size greater than 10 mm (12 mm in the sub-digastric area).

  → Central necrosis with heterogeneity and peripheral enhancement.

  → Circular shape

- MRI: to detect minimal neoplastic invasion to the cartilage. It is not routinely performed in staging of cancer of the larynx.
- Direct Pharyngo-laryngoscopy
- Goals: (1) multiple mucosal biopsies, (2) accurate evaluation of the tumour spread, (3) examination of the URT and the Esophagus for detection of synchronous cancers.
- U/S: for assessment of the cervical LN. It is a useful method for the follow-up and can be combined with FNA to confirm histological invasion.

Therapy

- Supraglottic SCC

- Supraglottic partial laryngectomy: for tumours limited to the epiglottis without extension to the pre-epiglottic space or involving the ventricle, minimal effect on voice, may require initial tracheotomy, postoperative swallowing therapy.
- Supracricoid partial laryngectomy with cricohyoidopexy: for a tumour extending to the inferior part of the pre-epiglottic space or involving the vocal cord or anterior commissure.
- External beam radiation: for patients with poor pulmonary function
- NECK: either RT or selective ND, both sides of the neck should be treated esp. for midline lesions.

- Glottic SCC

  A. Early laryngeal cancer (Stage I/II)
     - Mainly treated with single modality (either radiation or surgery)
     - Endoscopic laser excision or microlaryngeal traditional surgery
     - Radiotherapy
     - Involvement of anterior commissure: supracricoid partial laryngectomy.
     - NECK: low incidence of occult neck disease, no ND in N0 neck.
  B. Advanced cancer (Stage III/IV)
     - Concurrent chemoradiation for most T3 and early T4
     - Partial laryngectomy for selected cases (vertical partial laryngectomy, supracricoid laryngectomy with cricohyoidoepiglottopexy/CHEP)
     - Total laryngectomy with adjuvant RT for advanced T4
     - NECK: elective treatment of neck in N0 setting recommended in glottic T3 or T4 lesions. This can be completed with RT or ND with levels II–IV and VI.

3.23   Verrucous Carcinoma

- 1–2% of laryngeal carcinoma.
- Characterized by exophytic growth of well-differentiated keratinizing epithelium.
- Does not metastasize unless it has foci of conventional SCC.

Therapy

- Wide local surgical excision.
- No need for ND
- Radiation therapy not required.

3.24   Laryngeal Nerve Disorders

Etiology

- Lesions of brainstem
- Neurovascular disorders (stroke) and other central nervous disorders
- Demyelinating disorders of the peripheral nervous system (Guillain–Barré syndrome)
- Lateral skull-base lesions (trauma, tumour)
- Skull-base surgery
- Cervical spine injury or surgery
- Degenerative motor unit disorders (e.g. amyotrophic lateral sclerosis)
- Infectious diseases of the affected nerves
- Neurotoxins (e.g. lead)
- Primary neurogenic tumours (e.g. schwannoma)
- Malignant tumours of the thyroid, larynx, pharynx, trachea, oesophagus, bronchus, thymus, and other malignant tumours of the neck and mediastinum
- Traumatic lesions of the neck
- Aortic aneurysm

Symptoms

A. Unilateral paresis: hoarseness and breathiness of voice
B. Bilateral recurrent nerve paralysis: airway compromise

Diagnosis

- Detailed history (previous surgery, trauma)
- Indirect endoscopy with rigid and/or flexible scopes
- Stroboscopy
- Microlaryngoscopy, pharyngo-oesophagoscopy, and tracheobronchoscopy
- Voice analysis
- Thyroid gland workup (U/S, scintigraphy, TSH)
- Ultrasound of the neck
- CT scans of thorax and lateral skull base
- Barium swallow with fluoroscopy
- MRI studies of the brain (sign of neurogenic disorders)
- Pulmonary function test
- Laboratory tests
- Laryngeal electromyography

Therapy
Conservative

1. Unilateral VC paralysis
   - Initial voice rest
   - Oral steroids and non-steroidal antiphlogistics
   - Antiviral or antibiotic agents (if an infection is suspected)
   - Logopaedic treatment
2. Bilateral VC paralysis
   - Nasotracheal intubation for acute airway distress
   - High-dose intravenous steroids and non-steroidal antiphlogistics
   - Antiviral or antibiotic agents if an infection is suspected
   - Mild physical training once the patient has adjusted to the glottic narrowing
3. Deglutition disorders
   - Feeding via a nasogastric tube or PEG
   - Modifications in food consistency and viscosity
   - Postural manoeuvres to modify the flow of the bolus
   - Modifications in volume and tempo of food presentation

- Supraglottic swallow
- Exercises to increase muscle tone and to improve coordination

Surgical

1. Unilateral VC paralysis
   - Vocal fold augmentation using fat, collagen or dispersesilicone
   - Medialization thyroplasty using autologous cartilage or laryngeal implants
2. Bilateral VC paralysis
   - Temporary tracheotomy
   - Posterior cordectomy
   - Temporary or permanent laterofixation of one VC
   - Endoscopic arytenoidectomy
3. Deglutition disorders
   - Laryngeal elevation (thyrohyomandibulopexy)
   - Medialization thyroplasty (to reduce glottis gap)
   - Myotomy of the cricopharyngeal muscle

3.25   Laryngeal Trauma

Etiology: direct anterior blow with the head extended, strangulation.
- Nearly half of patients asphyxiate at the scene of the accident.
- In other cases airway obstruction develops after a fairly asymptomatic interval.

Symptoms

- Dyspnea and stridor.
- Dysphonia or aphonia.
- Cough and hemoptysis.
- Dysphagia and odynophagia.

Diagnosis

- Inspection
  - Neck hematoma

- Loss of neck contour due to flattening of thyroid cartilage.
- Subcutaneous emphysema
- Crepitus over laryngeal framework.

Therapy

Management is determined by stability of the airway:

- Acute airway distress:
  - urgent tracheotomy with local anesthesia, followed by direct laryngoscopy under general anesthesia to assess the injury.
- Stable airway:
  - Flexible laryngoscopy: to assess VF motion and look for lacerations and exposed cartilage.
    1. Normal: conservative management with observation, humidification and steroids.
    2. Hematoma, swelling, decreased motion → CT.
       If CT shows displaced fracture → surgical repair. Otherwise conservative management with steroids, observation, humidification.
    3. Lacerations or exposed cartilage: urgent tracheotomy with local anesthesia, followed by direct laryngoscopy under general anesthesia.
- Surgical repair: midline thyrotomy, lacerations should be sutured, defects should be closed with local flaps or free mucosal grafts. If an arytenoid is completely displaced, it is better to remove it.
- Laryngeal cartilage fractures should be reduced and immobilized (use of plates).

3.26 Laryngeal and Tracheal Stenosis

Etiology:

- trauma due to intubation or external injury
- systemic disease
- idiopathic

Symptoms

- Dyspnea
- Progressive stridor
- With or without hoarseness.

Diagnosis

- History: intubation or trauma
- Endoscopy: to evaluate supraglottic and glottis airway.
- CT: to evaluate subglottic and tracheal airway and crico-arytenoid joints.
- Direct laryngoscopy and bronchoscopy: to determine extent of lesion and palpate immobile vocal cords.

Therapy

- Supraglottic: endoscopic excision (often recurrence)
- External excision, supra-glottic laryngectomy (effective)
- Glottic (nearly always involves fixation of the VF due to posterior scarring): arytenoidectomy or cordotomy
- Subglottic: sometimes endoscopic excision (if the scar is thin and not circumferential)
- More often reconstructive surgery (either laryngotracheo-plasty or cricotracheal resection)
- Tracheal: resection and end-to-end anastomosis.
- Airway stenosis that involves multiple sites: difficult treatment, an option is a T-tube to stent the airway.

3.27   Aspiration of Foreign Body

The most common foods causing fatal aspiration are peanuts and grapes.

- Smaller objects do not cause complete airway obstruction.
- Foreign bodies that do not cause obstruction are present with wheezing and chronic cough.
- An observed choking event may be followed by an asymptomatic interval.
- Recurrent pneumonia (late manifestation).

Diagnosis

- Physical examination
  - tracheal: biphasic stridor
  - bronchial: expiratory wheeze, decreased breath sounds on involved side.
- Chest radiograph
  - only radiopaque foreign bodies are visible.
  - inspiratory and expiratory films show atelectasis on inspiration and hyperinflation on expiration on the affected side.
  - obstructive emphysema may be seen.

Therapy

- Removal by rigid ventilation bronchoscope.
  - Bronchoscopy indicated whenever diagnosis is suspected. All sign and symptoms need not be present.
  - General anesthesia is required with spontaneous ventilation.
  - Steroids are recommended to reduce edema.

Complications

1. bronchitis, pneumonia, ulceration, granulation tissue.
2. pneomothorax, pneumomediastinum.
3. vegetable matter may swell and become impacted.
4. total obstruction (as FB becomes lodged in larynx during removal).

Further Reading

1. Léauté-Labrèze C, Dumas de la Roque E, Hubiche T, Boralevi F, Thambo JB, Taïeb A. Propranolol for severe hemangiomas of infancy. N Engl J Med. 2008;358(24):2649–51.
2. Sand JP, Park AM, Bhatt N, Desai SC, Marquardt L, Sakiyama-Elbert S, Paniello RC. Comparison of conventional, revascularized, and bioengineered methods of recurrent laryngeal nerve reconstruction. JAMA Otolaryngol Head Neck Surg. 2016;142(6):526–32.

3. Lewis S, Earley M, Rosenfeld R, Silverman J. Systematic review for surgical treatment of adult and adolescent laryngotracheal stenosis. Laryngoscope. 2017;127(1):191–8.
4. Portnoy JE, Sataloff JB, Hawkshaw MJ, Sataloff RT. Arytenoid cartilage chondroma. Ear Nose Throat J. 2014;93(8):298.
5. Ludlow CL. Spasmodic dysphonia: a laryngeal control disorder specific to speech. J Neurosci. 2011;31(3):793–7.
6. Childs LF, Rickert S, Wengerman OC, Lebovics R, Blitzer A. Laryngeal manifestations of relapsing polychondritis and a novel treatment option. J Voice. 2012;26(5):587–9.
7. Steuer CE, El-Deiry M, Parks JR, Higgins KA, Saba NF. An update on larynx cancer. CA Cancer J Clin. 2017;67(1):31–50.

Chapter 4
Salivary Glands

4.1 Mumps

- The most common viral infection of the SGs.
- In 85% of cases it affects children (it also affects geriatric patients).
- Mumps is due to a paramyxovirus, an RNA virus related to influenza and parainfluenza virus.
- It is spread by aerosol droplets from the saliva and nasopharyngeal secretions.
- Incubation is from 2 to 3 weeks, and the patient is infectious 3 days before.
- Most children who present with an isolated acute, painful parotid swelling do not have mumps; similar symptoms scenarios can be caused by other viruses. These viral infections are not epidemic and are non-infectious, but are sporadic, and are commonly and erroneously labelled mumps. One can only be infected with the mumps virus once, because antibodies are precipitated during the initial infection, and this prevents any secondary infection.

Complications: orchitis, (25% in young males) pancreatitis, SNHL, meningoencephalitis, cause of abortion during the first trimester of pregnancy (fetal endocardial fibroelastosis).

P. Koltsidopoulos et al., *ENT*,
DOI 10.1007/978-3-319-56330-5_4,

Symptoms

– Unilateral or bilateral swelling
– The swelling lasts usually from a few days to 1 week.

Diagnosis

Stensen's papilla may be irritated and swollen, but no pus is visible or expressible.

Laboratory findings

– Leukocytopenia with relative lymphocytosis.
– Serum peaks the first week, and normalises at the second or third week.
– Soluble antibodies directed against the nucleoprotein core of the virus appear within the final week of infection, and disappear within 8 months.
– Antibodies directed against the outer surface appear several weeks after soluble antibodies do, and can persist for 5 years.

Therapy

– Antibiotics.
– Sialagogues
– Rehydration

The treatment depends on the clinical course and extent of the disease.

4.2   Acute Bacterial Sialadenitis

– The contamination mode of the parotid glands in cases of suppurative parotitis is unknown. Retrograde contamination of the gland by bacteria from the oral cavity, and stasis of salivary flow or reduced salivary flow might be the main causes.
– Coagulase-positive Staphylococcus is commonly encountered, but the flora is usually mixed (Streptococcus pneumonia, beta-haemolytic Streptococcus, gram-negative germs, anaerobic bacteria)

- Parotids are affected more frequently than are SMGs (bacteriostatic activity of the parotid saliva is inferior to that of the SMG saliva).
- Elderly patients are affected by marantic parotitis, caused by dehydration and poor oral hygiene.
- Small children can also be affected by this disease in the first 2 weeks of life (it affects premature infants, who are often dehydrated).

Symptoms

- Acute painful swelling of the salivary gland.
- Pressure over the affected gland elicits pain and purulent discharge at the papilla.

Therapy

- Massaging the gland and expressing pus and saliva—although painful—relieves the patient's pain by diminishing the pressure in the ductal system.
- Broad-spectrum antibiotics
- Anti-inflammatories
- Rehydration

In cases of severe infection and associated swelling and tautness of the skin, corticosteroids diminish inflammation and offer quick relief of symptoms.

4.3   Cat Scratch Disease

Pathogen: **Bartonella henselae**
 Reservoir for Bartonella is kittens; vector is cat flea

Symptoms

- Local lymphadenopathy; 10–30% spontaneously suppurates.
- Parinaud's oculoglandular syndrome: unilateral granulomatous conjunctivitis, associated with ipsilateral preauricular or submandibular lymphadenopathy.

Diagnosis

- History: exposure to cats, papule/pustule 1–2 weeks after exposure.
- Specific polymerase chain reaction (PCR) or serology.
- Cultures require 6-week incubation period.
- Test for antibodies to B. henselae

Therapy

The disease is self-limiting and the treatment is supportive. The affected LNs disappear spontaneously in 1–2 months.

4.4   Actinomycosis

Chronic suppurative infection that can occur in the head and neck region.

Pathogen: **Actinomycetes israelii**

- The disease is characterized by an abscess formation surrounded by a granulomatous inflammatory reaction.
- Drainage of pus
- Antibiotics (penicillin)

4.5   Sarcoidosis

Systemic inflammatory disease that manifests as non-caseating granulomas, primarily in the lungs and intra-thoracic lymph nodes.

- Unclear aetiology

Heerfort's disease (also called uveoparotid fever): rare form of sarcoidosis associated with parotid swelling, uveitis and facial palsy.

Symptoms

- Salivary Gs are usually affected, specifically the PG.
- Symptoms include swelling and xerostomia

Diagnosis

- Laboratory findings include diminishing amylase and kallikrein levels during the acute phase of the disease, and the presence of angiotensin-converting enzyme (ACE).
- Diagnosis is confirmed if there is radiologic and histologic evidence of non-caseous epithelial granulomas.
- Biopsy: non-caseous epithelial granulomas (obtained from minor salivary glands or the parotids).

Therapy

- Corticosteroids

4.6   HIV Pseudocysts

> Patients with HIV infection have been reported to develop lesions in the salivary glands such as lympho-epithelial cysts.

- They usually affect the PG.

Symptoms

- Soft, compressible, bilateral symmetric parotid swelling, especially if the parotid swelling appears multicystic.

Diagnosis

- CT scan or U/S
- FNA
- Serologic testing for HIV antibodies confirms the diagnosis.

Therapy

- repeated drainage
- Surgery
- Radiotherapy

4.7   Sialolithiasis

> Formation of salivary stones inside the ducts or parenchyma of salivary glands.

- The stones are composed of calcium and hydroxyapatite.
- It usually affects SMG (flow against gravity, more alkaline saliva, larger and longer duct).

  <u>Risk factors</u>: prolonged dehydration, gout, diabetes, hypertension, anti-cholinergic medication.

Symptoms

- Recurrent swelling
- Pain worse on eating

Diagnosis

- Inspection and palpation of the floor of the mouth
- U/S: the first line radiological
- Plain x-ray: most SMG stones are radio-opaque, most PG stones are radiolucent.
- MR sialography
- Sialography
- Sialendoscopy

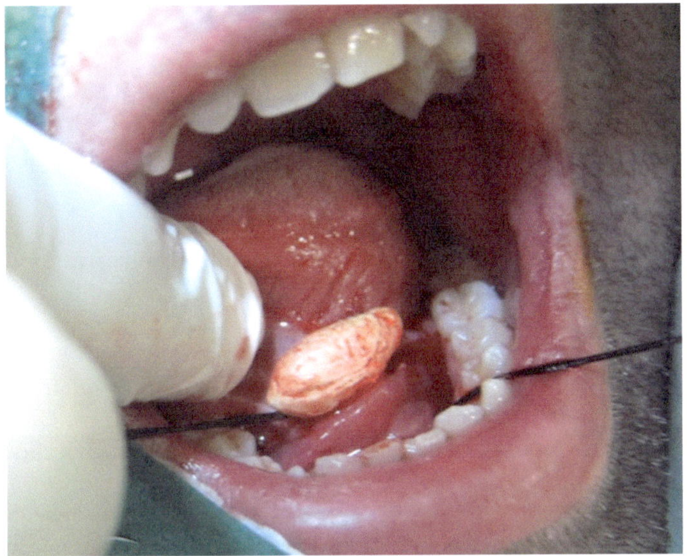

Therapy

- Intraoral extraction (stones near the duct orifice)
- Surgical excision of the gland (stones close to the gland)
- Interventional sialendoscopy
- External lithotripsy (effective in small stones)

4.8   Recurrent Parotitis in Children

- A rare, recurrent nonobstructive, and nonsuppurative parotid inflammation in young children.
- Its etiology remains unknown.
- Among aetiological factors considered are congenital malformations of the parotid ducts, familial history of the disease and impaired rates of secretion (primary or secondary infections, and local manifestations of systemic immunelogical disease).
- The most frequent non-viral infection of SGs in children.
- Age of presentation: from 8 months to 16 years, but more frequently from 5 to 7 years.

Symptoms

- It is characterized by recurrent episodes of swelling and or pain in the parotid gland usually associated with fever and malaise.
- It is usually unilateral, but bilateral exacerbation can also occur.
- Episodes recur every several months.
- The disease is self-limiting and usually resolves around puberty.

Diagnosis

- Inspection: Mucopurulent saliva can be expressed from the papilla, which is often erythematous.
- U/S: reveals typical diffuse oedema and a multiple hypoechogenic, polycystic appearance (pathognomonic)
- MR sialography without contrast medium: it primarily images liquid structures and the flow can be adequately demonstrated after stimulation with ascorbic acid.
- Sialendoscopy: reveals diffuse reduction of the calibre of Stensen's duct, associated sometimes with multiple localised stenoses, and rarely, salivary stones
- Histological appearance: massive infiltration with lymphocytes with lymph follicle formation and cystic ductal formations (sialectasis).

Therapy

- Anti-inflammatory medication.
- Antibiotics (in case of purulent discharge or persistent swelling despite anti-inflammatory treatment).

4.9   Mycobacteria

- Mycobacterium tuberculosis and atypical mycobacteria both affect LN adjacent to the SGs or the intraglandular tissue. Usually, they are contaminated by local infection affecting the mouth, the pharynx or the lungs.

Mycobacterium Tuberculosis
Symptoms: The clinical presentation can be an acute inflammatory lesion or achronic tumorous lesion.

Diagnosis: Purified protein derivative (PPD) skin test, which is then followed by FNA.

Therapy: Combination of antibiotics (Isoniazid, Rifampicin and Pyrazinamide).

Atypical Mycobacteria
In cases of atypical mycobacteria, both adults and infants can be infected; it is commonly seen in children between 2 and 5 years, and in adults suffering from immunodeficiency disorders.

Diagnosis: culture performed after therapeutic excisional biopsy of the lymph node, or by a specific PPD test. Its diagnosis is often delayed, as the classic PPD test remains negative.

Therapy: surgical excision, but sometimes curettage may eradicate the localised infection, depending on its location.

Chemotherapy may play a role in suboptimal surgery.

4.10 Sjoegren's Syndrome

> A systemic autoimmune disease of exocrine glands that presents with sicca symptomatology of the main mucosa surfaces.

– More common in perimeno-pausal Caucasian women.

Classification

Primary SS: it occurs in the absence of another underlying rheumatic disorder.
Associated SS: in association with another systemic auto-immune disease, most commonly rheumatoid arthritis (RA), systemic lupus erythematosus (SLE), or systemic sclerosis (SSc).

Symptoms

<u>Glandular Manifestations</u>

- Xerostomia ('95%)
- Xerophthalmia (ocular dryness)
- Diminished secretions from respiratory tract glands can lead to dryness of the nose, throat and trachea, resulting in persistent hoarseness and chronic, non-productive cough.
- Cutaneous dryness. In female patients, dryness of the vagina and vulva may result in pruritus and dyspareunia.
- Other oral symptoms:
  Difficulties in speaking, adherence of food to the mucosa, difficulties in eating dry food, local infections, tooth decay, periodontal disease and angular cheilitis.
- Other ocular symptoms: photosensitivity, erythema, eye fatigue or decreased visual acuity.
- Chronic or acute swelling of the major SGs (10–20%).

<u>Extraglandular symptoms</u>

- Primary SS: general symptoms, including fever, generalized pain, fatigue, weakness, sleep disturbances.
- Arthralgias
- Raynaud's phenomenon
- Involvement of internal organs
  - Pulmonary disease
  - Chronic pancreatitis.
  - Liver involvement.
  - Renal involvement (interstitial renal disease and glomerulo-nephritis).
- Peripheral neuropathy
- Psychiatric disorders (depression and anxiety).

Complications

- High incidence of lymphoma

Diagnosis

<u>Special Tests</u>

- Oral involvement
  - Measurement of the salivary flow rate, sialochemistry, sialography or scintigraphy.

- Ocular tests: Schirmer's test and rose Bengal staining.
- Minor SG biopsy (a highly specific test for the diagnosis of SS).

Focal lymphocytic sialadenitis, defined as multiple, dense aggregates of 50 or more lymphocytes in perivascular or periductal areas in the majority of sampled glands, is the characteristic histopathologic feature of SS. The key requirements for a correct histological evaluation are (1) an adequate number of informative lobules (at least four) and the (2) determination of an average focus score (a focus is a cluster of at least 50 lymphocytes).

<u>Laboratory Findings</u>

- The most frequent findings are cytopenia (33%), increased erythrocyte sedimentation rate (22%) and hypergammaglobulinaemia (22%).
- The most frequent cytopenia is normocytic anaemia (20%), leucopoenia (16%) and thrombocytopenia (13%).
- Immunological markers found in primary SS:
  - Antinuclear antibodies ANA, ('80% of cases), titres >1/80.
  - Anti-Ro/SS-A and La/SS-B antibodies (30–60%).
  - Rheumatoid factor (50%).
  - Hypocomplementaemia and cryoglobulinaemia have been linked with more severe SS.
  - Circulating monoclonal immunoglobulins (20%).

Therapy

- Symptomatic replacement or stimulation of glandular secretions, while extraglandular involvement requires an organ-specific therapy with steroids and immune-suppressive agents.
- Treatment of xerostomia
  - Sipping fluids, chewing sugar-less gum, using artificial saliva.
  - For patients with residual SG function: secretagogues (pilocarpine and cevimeline).
  - Avoidance of anticholinergic medications, alcohol and smoking.

- Oral hygiene and regular dental visits.
- Prompt removal of salivary stones.
- Pain of suddenly enlarged salivary glands is treated with warm compresses and NSADs.
- Treatment of ocular manifestations
  - Tear substitutes, lubricating ointments.
- Treatment of systemic manifestations
  - It should be organ specific, with steroids and immune-suppressive agents being limited to severe involvement.
  - NSAIDs for minor musculoskeletal symptoms.
  - Hydroxychloroquine is used in patients with fatigue, arthralgias and myalgias.
  - For patients with moderate extra-glandular involvement (mainly arthritis, extensive cutaneous purpura and non-severe peripheral neuropathy), steroids may be sufficient.
  - For patients with internal organ involvement: prednisone and immunosuppressive agents.
  - A promising treatment is rituximab (anti-CD20).

4.11   Sialosis

Characterized by persistent, asymptomatic, bilateral, diffuse, non-inflammatory, non-neoplastic parotid swelling with occasional involvement of the submandibular salivary gland and, rarely, the minor salivary glands.

Sialosis is related to four main conditions:

1. Idiopathic
2. Nutritional
   (a) Malnutrition
   (b) Bulimia
   (c) Gastrointestinal disease
   (d) Amylophagia
   (e) Vitamin A deficiency

3. Drug induced
   (a) Alcohol
   (b) Antihypertensives
   (c) Naproxen
   (d) Valproic acid
4. Endocrine/metabolic
   (a) Diabetes insipidus
   (b) Diabetes mellitus
   (c) Hypothyroidism
   (d) Cirrhosis of the liver
   (e) Uraemia

Diagnosis

- Clinical history
- Physical examination
  - The groove between the mastoid process and the ramus of the mandible becomes obliterated.
- Palpation of PGs and SMGs
- Blood analyses
  - Study of liver enzymes, bilirubin, protein and albumin levels
- CT scan, searching any intraglandular lesions or calcified bodies
- MRI for excluding other diseases (the best image test for SGs study)
- FNA biopsy
  - Swelling could be associated with benign acinic cells and adipose tissue but no inflammatory or abnormal cells.
- Sialography
  - There is a lack of arborisation being caused by the separation of secretory ducts from each other and compression of smaller interlobular canaliculi.

Treatment

Treatment of sialosis is unnecessary.

4.12   Benign Tumours of Salivary Glands

- 70–85% of SG neoplasms originate in the PG, 10% SMG, 10% MSG.
- The majority (80–85%) of PG tumours is benign, and the rate decreases for the SMG (40–55%), minor salivary glands (MSG; 20–50%) and sublingual gland (SLG; 15–30%).
- Pleomorphic adenoma (PA) is most frequently encountered (about 60% of all salivary gland tumours.

Lesions in the Superficial Lobe

- A slow-growing, painless lesion in the preauricular or retro-mandibular areas.
- The mass usually shows well-defined margins; at palpation, it may appear mobile over superficial and deep planes, with firm or hard consistency.

Lesions in the Deep Lobe

- The lesion is barely palpable. Medialisation of the lateral oro-pharyngeal wall and/or the soft palate may be observed (dysphagia and/or dyspnea).

Lesions in the Accessory Lobe

- A midcheek mass with the same physical features of a lesion of the superficial lobe. Submandibular Gland
- A slow-growing, painless mass in the submandibular region.

Sublingual Gland

- Slow-growing, painless, submucosal mass in the anterior floor of the mouth, lateral to the lingual caruncle.
- It may cause discomfort in lingual movements and during speech.
- SLG benign tumours are rare, and any lesion in this area should be considered malignant until proven otherwise.

Minor Salivary Glands

- Slow-growing, painless, submucosal mass in any head and neck region (sinonasal tract, oral cavity, pharynx, larynx, trachea and parapharyngeal space).
- Oral cavity and oropharynx are the most frequently involved sites.
- Superficial ulceration is seldom observed in benign tumours of MSG.
- According to the site of origin, different complaints may be present:
    - Sinonasal tract: nasal obstruction, recurrent sinusitis
    - Nasopharynx: otitis media due to tube compression
    - Oropharynx: dysphagia
    - Larynx: dyspnea, hoarseness
    - Trachea: dyspnea

Diagnosis

- Inspection of scalp and skin of the pre-auricular region.
- Inspection of the oral cavity, floor of mouth and oropharynx.
- Palpation of the gland and ipsilateral neck LN (levels I–V)
- Palpation of contralateral gland and neck LN.
- Evaluation and palpation of major salivary gland excretory ducts (Stensen's, Wharton's), with and without concomitant compression on the relative gland.
- Ultrasonography (US) of the SG and of the ipsi-lateral neck LN, better if combined with US-guided fine-needle aspiration cytology (FNAC) or core biopsy as a first step;
- US should also include the contralateral gland and LN, especially when there is risk for bilateral involvement (WT)
- MRI (or CT with contrast when MRI is not feasible) (1) when dealing with lesions with critical extension, deep lobe or parapharyngeal space involvement, (2) recurrent disease after previous surgery or (3) clinically suspicious for malignancy.

- SL tumours: should be evaluated by CT or MRI, due to their limited visibility at US, and to define better their local extension.
- When a MSG lesion is suspected:
  - Endoscopic evaluation of the involved site of onset.
  - An imaging study (CT and/or MRI) to better evaluate local extension of the lesion should be performed.
  - Biopsy under local anaesthesia.

Therapy
Surgery

- Parotid Gland
  - Lesion limited to the superficial lobe: superficial (or lateral) parotidectomy or extracapsular dissection.
  - Lesion involving or arising within the accessory lobe: superficial parotidectomy anteriorly extended
  - Lesion involving the deep lobe: total parotidectomy
- Submandibular Gland
  - Submandibular gland excision
- Sub-lingual Gland
  - Sublingual gland excision
- Minor Salivary Gland
  - Wide excision of the lesion according the site of origin

Pleomorphic adenoma

1. PA originates within the PG in about 80% of cases, whereas the remaining 20% occur in the SMG and MSG.
2. Tendency to recur
3. Potential for malignant degeneration into carcinoma ex PA (5–10%)
   - Malignant degeneration should be suspected whenever a SG mass:
     - has a rapid growth
     - gives rise to complaints like pain
     - facial nerve palsy
     - LN swelling

Histologic characteristics:

- Presence of a so-called pseudocapsule.
- Finger-like tumour projections extending into the parenchyma.
- Treatment of recurrent PA quite challenging, due to:
  - the complexity of revision surgery,
  - the high risk of facial nerve lesions and
  - the risk of further recurrences.

Warthin tumor

- Malignant degeneration is exceedingly rare (about 1%)
- WT is multicentric (synchronous or metachronous) in up to 20 % of cases, with bilateral involvement in up to 15% of patients.

4.13   Malignant Salivary Glands Neoplasms

A. Primary neoplasm: A malignant tumor of a major SG.
B. Secondary neoplasm:
   1. Lymphatic metastases to LN within the SG of a tumor of other origin,
   2. Haematogenous metastases from distant primary tumors or
   3. Direct invasion from tumors that are located adjacent to the SG.

Negative prognostic factors: facial palsy, initial pain, LN metastases, cancer of minor SGs, advanced stage, high grade tumors, positive surgical margins (R+), perineural spread.

Symptoms

Parotid Glands

- Facial palsy (most probably incomplete)
- Pain
- Skin infiltration
- Cervical adenopathy

Submandibular Glands

– Weakness or numbness of the tongue (spread along the hypoglossal or the lingual nerve).
– Pain
– Skin infiltration
– Fixation to the mandible (signs of local extension)

Minor Salivary Glands

– Presentation depends on the site of the tumor
– The palate is the most common site, and the tumor usually manifests as a submucosal mass or ulceration. The second most common site is the sinonasal tract.

Diagnosis

- Inspection
  - red, prominent auricle
  - swollen skin over the mastoid
  - facial palsy
- Inspection of the skin of head and neck
  - possible skin cancer
- Inspection of the oral cavity and the neck
- Palpation
  - painful, fixed or mobile tumor
  - skin infiltration
- Palpation of the neck
  - possible metastases
- Otoscopy in cases of parotid tumors: possible infiltration of the ear canal.
- U/S of major SG and neck
- FNA cytology
- MRI of neck: evaluation of the extent of the disease, esp. for deep-lobe parotid tumors or those with para-pharyngeal extension.
- CT of the neck: possible bone infiltration
- Tumor staging using the tumor-node-metastasis (TNM) system.

- X-ray of the chest: staging procedure.
- MRI of abdomen: in cases of secondary neoplasm.
- Electrodiagnostics of facial n.: in cases of facial palsy.
- 18FDG-PET: of limited value in comparison to CT and MRI, but superior in distinguishing tumor recurrence from post-treatment fibrosis during follow-up.
- Frozen section: should be reserved for cases where FNA was not possible, or the results were unclear.
  [Note: sensitivity and specificity of frozen sections is less than that of FNA cytology].

Therapy

- Non-resectable tumors: RT (fast neutron R) alone or CRT (platinum based)
- Resectable tumors: Complete surgical excision and adjuvant RT or CRT.

Surgical treatment

<u>Parotid tumors</u>

- Lateral parotidectomy: T1/T2
- Total parotidectomy: larger tumors and all deep-lobe tumors
- Radical parotidectomy (facial n. resection).
- Extended parotidectomy: tumor extending beyond the PG (including skin, soft tissue, masseter muscle resection, infratemporal fossa dissection, mastoidectomy or even petrosectomy).

<u>Submandibular tumors</u>

- Small tumors: resection of the gland
- Advanced tumors: wide en block resection of submandibular triangle, and may need resection of the floor of the mouth, mylohyoid and digastric muscles, or segmental/ marginal mandibulectomy.
  - Infiltration and consecutive thickening of the lingual, hypoglossal, mylohyoid or marginal mandibular nerve indicate resection of the involved nerves.

<u>Minor salivary gland tumors</u>

- Oral cavity: small tumors are treated by wide local excision; advanced tumors require radical excision with segmental/marginal mandibulectomy, or partial maxillectomy.
- Sinonasal tract: usually high grade tumors that need partial or total maxillectomy.

Infiltration of the second (V2) or third (V3) branch of the trigeminal nerve are managed by nerve resection, as these nerves provide a route to skull base invasion.

<u>Treatment of the neck</u>:

- Evidence of neck metastases (N+): ND is performed (selective, modified or radical).
- Negative for neck metastases (N0): It is unclear in which cases do patients profit from elective ND. Recent studies report occult metastasis rates as much as 25–40% independent of the histological subtype. Older reports recommend ND only for high-grade tumors. The highest occult metastasis rate is seen in advanced stages (T3/T4).

4.14   Frey's Syndrome

- Less than 5% of patients after parotidectomy.
- 6–12 months after surgery
- Aberrant regeneration of the parasympathetic fibres that normally innervate the PG (they are redirected to the sweat glands).

<u>Minor's iodine-starch test</u>:

1. Patient's face on the affected side is painted with an iodine solution, which is allowed to dry for 1–2 min.
2. The entire area is dusted with starch powder.
3. Patient eats a sialogogue (lemon slice, aplle) to evoke gustatory stimulation.
4. Typically, within 5 min, the starch turns blue in the area where saliva is produced.

Therapy: Botulinum toxin injection.

Further Reading

1. Sujatha D, Babitha K, Prasad RS, Pai A. Parotid lymphoepithelial cysts in human immunodeficiency virus: a review. J Laryngol Otol. 2013;127(11):1046–9.
2. Capaccio P, Sigismund PE, Luca N, Marchisio P, Pignataro L. Modern management of juvenile recurrent parotitis. J Laryngol Otol. 2012;126(12):1254–60.
3. Seror R, Theander E, Bootsma H, Bowman SJ, Tzioufas A, Gottenberg JE, Ramos-Casals M, Dörner T, Ravaud P, Mariette X, Vitali C. Outcome measures for primary Sjögren's syndrome: a comprehensive review. J Autoimmun. 2014;51:51–6.
4. Mendenhall WM, Mendenhall CM, Werning JW, Malyapa RS, Mendenhall NP. Salivary gland pleomorphic adenoma. Am J Clin Oncol. 2008;31(1):95–9.
5. Motz KM, Kim YJ. Auriculotemporal syndrome (Frey syndrome). Otolaryngol Clin North Am. 2016;49(2):501–9.

Chapter 5
Neck

5.1 Thyroglossal Cyst

> Remnants of thyroglossal duct, which normally obliterates by the end of the 8th embryonic week and become completely reabsorbed.

- It can occur anywhere along the developmental path of the thyroid gland. However, the majority occur in the proximity of the hyoid bone.
- Up to 20% of the lesions have been reported to contain thyroid tissue.

Symptoms

- Midline swelling in neck with intermittent increase in swelling and pain due to infections.
- Dysphagia and dyspnea (large cysts).

Diagnosis

- Inspection
    - Recurrent supralaryngeal cystic, swelling, 1–3 cm in size, painless and non-tender.
    - Depending on the size, protrusion of the tongue is possible.

P. Koltsidopoulos et al., *ENT*,
DOI 10.1007/978-3-319-56330-5_5,
© Springer International Publishing AG 2017

- The mass moves with tongue protrusion.
- In 10–15% of cases infection can occur (reddening, pain).

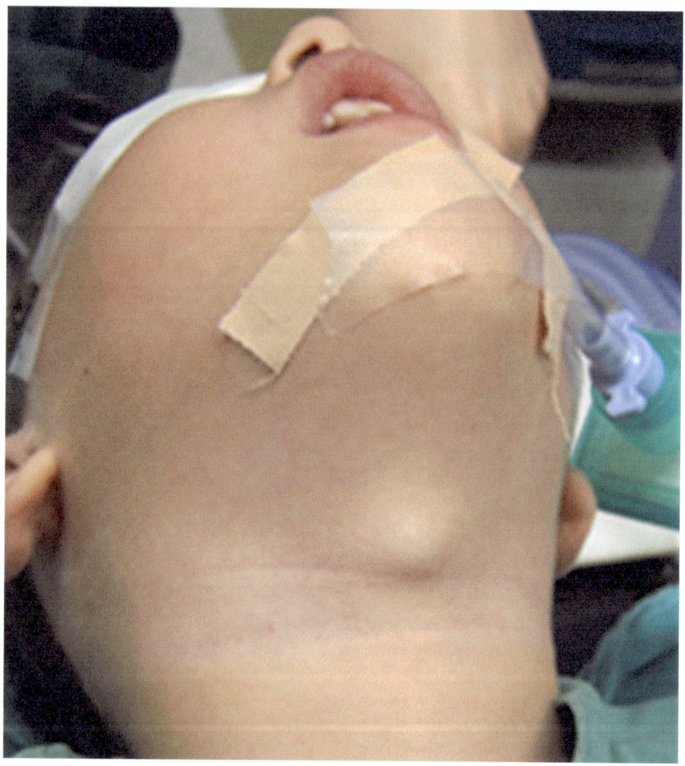

- Palpation
  - Bimanual palpation of the floor of mouth and tongue
- Endoscopy of hypo-pharynx: to identify foramen caecum
- FNA

Therapy

Surgical removal
- Sistrunk procedure: it includes excision of the thyroglossal duct cyst, its tract, and the body of the hyoid bone.

- If the middle portion of the hyoid bone is not resected, there is a high risk of recurrence.
- If the epithelial trunk continues cranially, it must be followed up to the tongue base.

D/D
- Enlarged lymph node
- Dermoid cyst
- Ectopic thyroid tissue
- Plunging ranula

5.2   Dermoid Cyst

> Squamous epithelial-lined cavities that contain dermal adnexal structures such as sebaceous glands, hair follicles, or sweat glands in the cyst wall.

Common sites:

- Periorbital (most common site)
- Nasal (frontonasal suture and rhinion)
- Intraoral (floor of mouth),
- Scalp (anterior fontanelle and cranial sutures)
- Postauricular.

Diagnosis

- Mass is non-tender, non-compressible and firm.
- CT and MRI: important for determining extent of lesion.

Therapy

- Surgical removal

5.3   Ranula

> A ranula is a mucocele of the floor of the mouth, arising from an isolated accessory salivary gland, or from the sublingual gland.

Classification:

1. Simple ranula: confined to the oral cavity
2. Plunging ranula: extends through the fibers of the mylohyoid muscle in the anterior neck.

Symptoms

- Painless, fluctuant, with a blue translucent color swelling, and slowly growing mass of the floor of the mouth.

Diagnosis

- It is generally based on the clinical examination.
- Imaging (ultrasonography, computed tomography scanning, and magnetic resonance imaging): to determine the size and the location of the lesion. An MRI scan is considered a gold standard.

Therapy

- Surgical removal of the entire cyst, and it might include in some cases the entire sublingual gland to avoid recurrences.

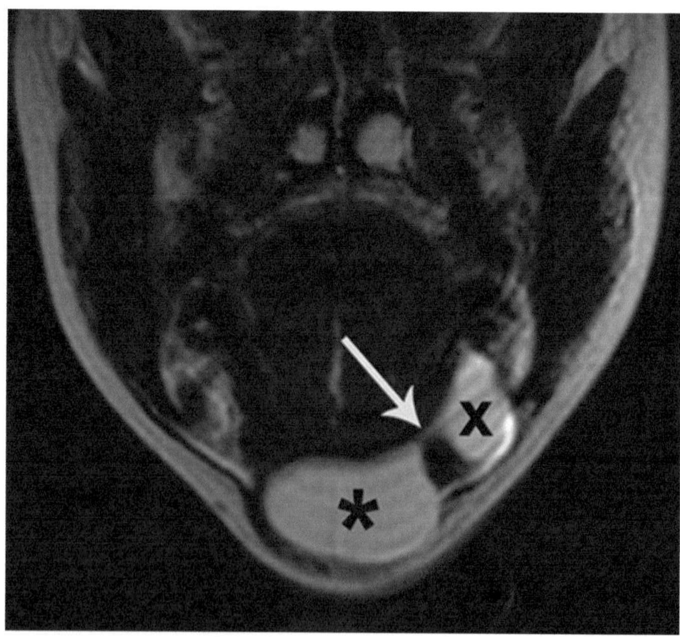

5.4   Branchial Cyst

Branchial cleft defects can manifest as cysts, sinuses, or fistulas. Branchial clefts are categorized into first, second, and third branchial cleft defects, depending on the location of the defect.

The second branchial cleft cyst/fistula is the most common.

Classification

- *First branchial cleft cyst/fistula*: located either in the preauricular region usually anterior to the pinna, or posterior to or inferior to the angle of the mandible.
- *Second branchial cleft cyst*: found along the anterior border of the SCM muscle. The tract passes over the bifurcation of the carotid artery, and between the ECA and ICA, and enters the lateral wall of the pharynx at the tonsillar fossa.
- Third *branchial cleft cyst*: along the anterior border of SCM. The tract passes laterally to the CCA, posteriorly to the ICA and deviates medially, and finally opens at the pyriform sinus.
- Fourth *branchial cleft cyst/fistula*: It begins at the apex of the pyriform sinus and exits the pharynx caudally to the superior laryngeal nerve, the cricothyroid muscle and the thyroid cartilage. These fistulae open to the skin anteriorly to the lower portion of SCM muscle.

Diagnosis

- Inspection: well-visible mass, often of changing size and feelings of pressure.
- Palpation: bimanual palpation of the lateral neck cyst together with the ipsilateral tonsil. Is there a common mobility?
- Exploration of a fistula with a probe.
- U/S: to find out if the lesion is solid or fluid filled
- FNA
- MRI with contrast

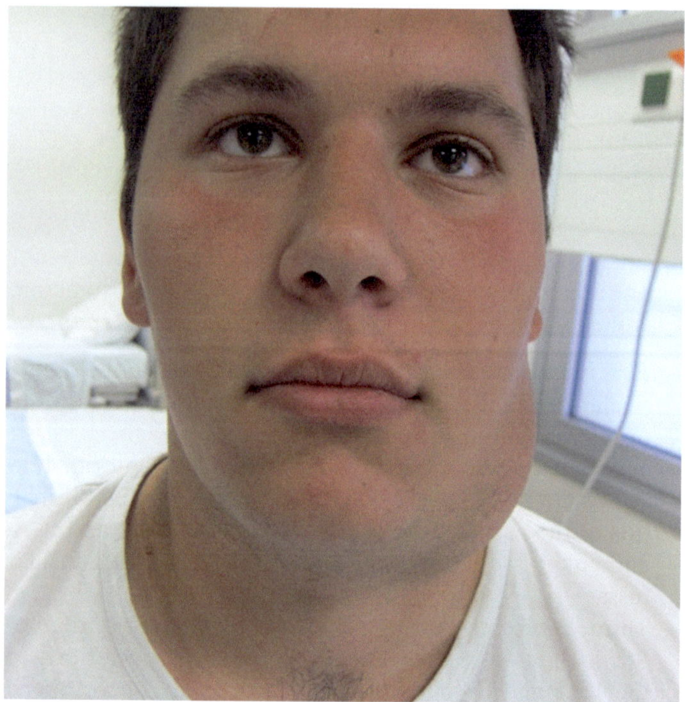

Complications

- Abscess
- Branchiogenic carcinoma (patients older than 40 years)

Therapy

- Complete surgical excision
- The cyst and the entire fistula must be resected to avoid recurrences.

D/D

- Unspecific or specific lymphadenopathy
- Metastatic carcinoma in cervical lymph nodes
- Malignant lymphoma

- Paraganglioma
- Haemangioma
- Lymphangioma
- Dermoid cyst
- Laryngocele

5.5   Hemangioma

> Self-limiting vascular tumors evolving a few weeks after birth.

- The most common vascular tumor in children.
- Around 85% of all infantile haemangiomas manifest themselves in the first few weeks of life.

Phases of the life cycle of hemangiomas

1. Proliferative (rapid growth from 2 weeks to 1 year),
2. Involuting (slow regression, 1–8 years),
3. Involuted (complete regression after 8 years of age).
   - The mechanism that controls the involution of hemangiomas is still unknown.
   - Approximately 50% of infantile haemangiomas are resolved by 5 years of age, and 70% by 7 years of age.

Diagnosis

- Inspection
  - A haemangioma presents as a skin lesion or cystic mass.
  - The size of the lesion changes when the child strains or cries.
  - The lesion is compressible, and causes surrounding skin to appear bluish.
- MRA
- CT: not always characteristic.
- FNA confirms the diagnosis

Therapy

1. Observation (wait and see strategy)
2. Treatment is indicated:
    A. If the hemangioma causes symptoms by pressure on adjacent structures (visual compromise, airway obstructive, congestive heart failure)
    B. Aesthetic considerations (permanent disfigurement)
    C. Ulceration, bleeding

<u>Treatment options</u>

- Sclerotherapy (intralesional steroid or interferon a injection).
- Systemic steroids
- Propranolol: can effectively control the proliferation of severe hemangioma and promote its regression
- Subcutaneous injection of interferon a-2a or 2b
- Laser therapy (argon laser, pulsed dye laser and Nd: YAG laser etc.)
- Surgical resection

5.6   Lymphangioma

Congenital malformation of lymphatic channels.

- The majority of these lesions occur in the neck.

<u>Classification</u>

1. Lymphangioma simplex (capillary-sized, thin-walled lymphatics)
2. Cavernous lymphangioma (dilated lymphatic spaces)
3. Cystic hygroma (lymphatic cysts ranging from a few mm to several cm in diameter).
    - Lymphangioma presents with similar symptoms as haemangiomas. However, it can become very extensive and infiltrate the soft tissues of the neck and oral cavity.

- Lymphatic malformations are usually present in infancy, with 90% being detected before 2 years of age.

Diagnosis

- Clinical examination
- Ultrasound
- CT scan and/or MRI
- FNA confirms the diagnosis

Therapy

- Surgical resection
- Sclerotherapy
- Incision and drainage
- Aspiration
- Radiation therapy

5.7   Chronic Lymph Node Diseases

- Caused by both bacteria and viruses.
- Diseases associated with chronic lymphadenopathy: toxoplasmosis, cat scratch disease, tularaemia, brucellosis and sarcoidosis.
- The most common causes for chronic LN disease are nowadays due to atypical mycobacteria, Mycobacterium tuberculosis and HIV.
- FNA: can aid in diagnosis.
- If this is not conclusive, the entire LN should be removed.

Atypical Mycobacteria infection
- Found in children who have not received vaccination against tuberculosis.
- Atypical Mycobacteria are resistant to antibiotics and chemotherapeutics
- Enlarged LN and eventually fixation of it to the overlying skin, which can become inflamed.
- Sometimes spontaneous fistulation takes place.
- Excision of the LN (at times including some overlying skin), or to perform curettage to remove the infected tissue.

Tuberculosis
- Neck involvement often occurs simultaneously with pulmonary disease.
- The affected LN can be found anywhere along the jugular lymph node chain, but usually are along its caudal region and the posterior fossa.
- Diagnosis is confirmed by FNA
- An open LN extirpation might be necessary.
- A chest X-ray is essential.
- Further handling is outside the scope of otorhinolaryngology.

5.8   Cervical Necrotizing Fasciitis

Rapid spreading disease of the soft tissue, which includes the superficial fascia and subcutaneous layer of tissue.

- Risk factors: diabetes mellitus, elderly, acute, or chronic renal disease, postpartum period, alcoholism, intravenous (IV) drug use, malnutrition, malignancy, peripheral vascular disease, and radiation exposure.
- Etiologic factors: dental infections (commonest), trauma, peritonsillar abscess, osteoradionecrosis, infections of the tonsils or the pharynx, injury, foreign bodies, cervical adenitis, surgical wounds, and tumors.
- The infection tends to spread to all fasciae and muscle tissues in the neck.
- Mixed aerobic and anaerobic flora.

Symptoms

- Diffuse spreading erythematous pitting neck edema with "orange-peel" appearance secondary to obstructed dermal lymphatics.

Diagnosis

- Subcutaneous crepitus.

- CT neck with contrast: cervical subcutaneous gas in 50% of cases, diffuse loculated hypodense areas without rim

Therapy
<u>If necrotizing fasciitis is not treated early, it is potentially a fatal disease</u>

- Broad-spectrum IV antibiotics
- Airway securement
- Surgical excision of necrotic tissues and opening of all fasciae for decompression.
- Adjuvant hyperbaric oxygen.

Prognosis: mortality of 20–30% in treated patients

5.9   Cervical Vagal Schwannoma

> A benign, slow-growing mass, often asymptomatic, with a very low lifetime risk of malignant transformation.

Symptoms

- Mass in lateral neck
- Pain and neurologic dysfunctions are rare.
- Hoarseness: the most common specific symptom due to vocal cord palsy

Diagnosis

- Clinical: a slow-growing asymptomatic mass, well circumscribed and encapsulated, having an enlargement rate of 2.5–3 mm per year.
- Paroxysmal cough during palpation of the mass due to vagal stimulation: pathognomonic sign for vagal schwannoma.
- FNA: helpful
- MRI or CT scan: to assess the extent of the lesion.

<u>Differential diagnosis from schwannoma:</u>

- Paraganglioma
- Branchial cleft cyst
- Inflammatory adenopathies
- Malignant lymphoma
- Metastatic cervical lymphoadenopathies
- Submandibular salivary gland tumours
- Carotid artery aneurysm

Therapy

– Surgical resection (with an attempt to preserve the integrity of the nerve origin).
– Debulking: a valuable treatment as there is a risk of malignant transformation (developing into sarcomas).
– Post-operative complications: ipsilateral vocal cord palsy.

5.10   Paraganglioma (Glomus Caroticum)

Benign neuroendocrine tumor arising from carotid body paraganglia.

- Normal function of carotid body is as a chemo-receptor for changes in blood oxygen, carbon dioxide and hydrogen ion concentration.
- Sites of predilection: carotid bifurcation, vagal nerve, larynx and temporal bone.
- Multiple localizations occur in the neck in 15–20% of cases
- Sporadic: most common, in fifth and sixth decades, rarely bilateral (5%)
- Familial: at a younger age, less likely to be malignant, increased incidence of bilaterality (30%) and multilocality.
- Hyperplastic: due to chronic hypoxia, in populations living at higher altitudes.

- May encase carotid (Shamblin classification)
    I. small tumor, easily separated from carotid.
    II. tumor partially encircles carotid and is difficult to separate.
    III. tumor completely encircles carotid and is densely adherent.
- Malignancy is rare (5–10%)
    - pain is the most predictive feature, along with young age and rapid enlargement.
- Rarely functional (1–3%)
    - if history of hypertension or flushing, consider workup for catecholamine byproducts (plasma free metanephrines, 24-h urine fractionated metanephrines).

Diagnosis

- Physical examination
    - Slow growing deep neck mass high in the neck.
    - Tethered vertically but mobile horizontally (Fontaine sign).
    - May be pulsatile or have a bruit.
- Contrast-enhanced CT
    - hypervascular mass typically splaying ICA and ECA.
        1. If mass pushes both vessels anteromedially a vagal tumor is considered.
        2. If mass pushes vessels laterally → sympathetic tumor.
        3. If mass is located above the bifurcation, an entity other than a carotid body tumor should be expected.
    - halo between carotid and tumor suggests a good plane of separation.
- MRI: "salt and pepper" appearance.
- Angiography: "lyre sign", splaying of ICA and ECA by vascular mass. Useful if preoperative embolization planned.
- FNA to be avoided, core-needle or open biopsy to be condemned.

Therapy

A. Surgical excision
   - For small tumors in healthy patients.
   - Preoperative embolization significantly reduces surgical blood loss.
   - COMP: cranial n. X and XII injured, first bite syndrome (parotid pain on initiate eating due to injury of cervical sympathetics), baroreflex failure (tachycardia and blood pressure lability due to loss of carotid sinus reflex)
B. Radiation therapy:
   - For unresectable cases, or poor operative candidates.
   - Tumors do not regress, but remain stable.
   - Postoperative RT should be considered for metastatic cases.

5.11   Glomus Vagale (Vagal Paraganglioma)

Paragangliomas involving the vagus nerve ganglia is termed glomus vagale.

- They account for 5–9% of all the head and neck paragangliomas.
- Have a higher incidence of malignancy than carotid body tumors.
- Typically arise from the inferior ganglion but can arise from middle or superior ganglion.

Symptoms

- Preoperative weakness of CN X occurs in one-third of patients.

Diagnosis

Contrast-enhanced CT or MRI
- Vascular tumor typically displacing both external and internal carotid arteries anteromedially without splaying.
- Vagal tumors tend to separate the jugular vein from the carotid sheath, whereas sympathetic tumors do not.

Therapy

<u>Surgical resection</u>
- essentially guarantees vagal paralysis.
- used for aggressive tumors invading the skull base and for patients with preexisting vagal paralysis.
- cervical approach for lower tumors and lateral skull base approach for higher tumors.

<u>Radiation therapy or observation</u>
- for patients with small tumors and no preexisting vagal weakness.

Further Reading

1. Righini CA, Hitter A, Reyt E, Atallah I. Thyroglossal duct surgery. Sistrunk procedure. Eur Ann Otorhinolaryngol Head Neck Dis. 2016;133(2):133–6.
2. Morton RP, Ahmad Z, Jain P. Plunging ranula: congenital or acquired? Otolaryngol Head Neck Surg. 2010;142(1):104–7.
3. Bradley PT, Bradley PJ. Branchial cleft cyst carcinoma: fact or fiction? Curr Opin Otolaryngol Head Neck Surg. 2013;21(2):118–23.
4. Adams MT, Saltzman B, Perkins JA. Head and neck lymphatic malformation treatment: a systematic review. Otolaryngol Head Neck Surg. 2012;147(4):627–39.
5. King E, Chun R, Sulman C. Pediatric cervicofacial necrotizing fasciitis: a case report and review of a 10-year national pediatric database. Arch Otolaryngol Head Neck Surg. 2012;138(4):372–5.

6. Mafee MF, Raofi B, Kumar A, Muscato C. Glomus faciale, glomus jugulare, glomus tympanicum, glomus vagale, carotid body tumors, and simulating lesions. Role of MR imaging. Radiol Clin North Am. 2000;38(5):1059–76.

Chapter 6
Carcinomas

6.1 Carcinoma of the Lip

- Most common site for cancer of the oral cavity.

Types: (1) SCC (95%), (2) Minor salivary gland carcinomas, (3) BCCs
Location: 95% lower lip, 5% upper lip
Risk factors: sunlight exposure, tobacco

Symptoms

Early: blistering, crusting, ulceration, or leukoplakia
Late: mandibular invasion, involvement of mental nerve.
Diagnosed early because of prominent location.

Metastases

- Regional metastases in 10% of patients
- Occur later in the course of disease as compared to other oral cavity sites.
- Lymphatic drainage is primarily to submental and sub-mandibular nodes.

Therapy

- Small lesions (T1, T2): either RT or surgery only.
- Large lesions (T3, T4): combined therapy.

P. Koltsidopoulos et al., *ENT*,
DOI 10.1007/978-3-319-56330-5_6,

- Postoperative radiation therapy is indicated in high-risk patients.
    - locally advanced disease (T3–T4)
    - perineural invasion
    - positive margins
    - multiple LN metastases
- Neck dissection: for clinically apparent lymphadenopathy.

Reconstruction

- Reconstruction is based on the size of the defect.
- Proper alignment of vermilion border is critical.

6.2   Carcinoma of the Oral Tongue

- Second most common site for cancer of the oral cavity.
- Most often along the lateral borders.

<u>Risk factors</u>: tobacco, alcohol, immunosuppression.
High risk patients (higher rates of metastasis, recurrence and mortality):

- depth of tumor invasion >2–4 mm
- perineural invasion

Symptoms

Early: Erythroplakia (the most common form of early SCC).
Late: tongue fixation, decreased tongue sensation, alteration in speech and swallowing, cervical lymphadenopathy.

Metastases

- Drainage to levels I–III
- Incidence depends on size of tumor and depth of invasion (clinically detectable 25–33%)

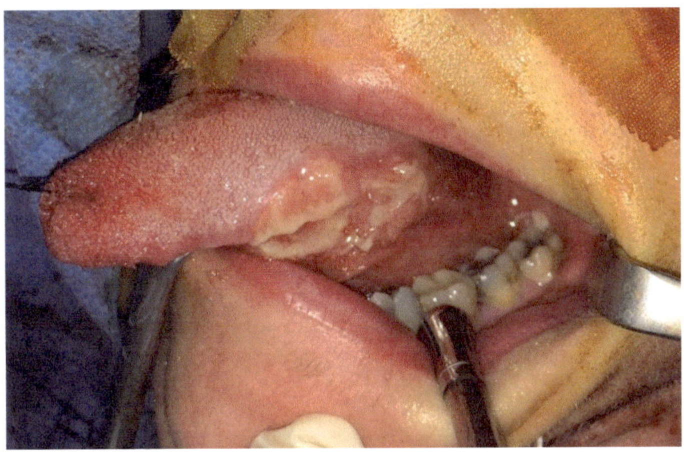

Therapy

A. Management of primary
  - T1–T2: partial glossectomy or radiation (in patients not suitable for surgery).
  - Extensive local disease: near-total or total glossectomy (difficult reconstruction)
  - T4: CRT
B. Management of mandible
  - tumors extending superficially to the gingival require resection with periosteum.
  - tumors involving periosteum require marginal mandibulectomy
  - direct bone invasion → segmental mandibulectomy.
C. Management of neck
  - Level I–III (supraomohyoid) treatment of neck for tumors with depth of invasion > 2–4 mm.
  - Bilateral ND should be performed for midline cancers.
  - Sentinel LN biopsy is accurate for staging the regional lymphatics in patients with T1–T2/N0 oral cavity cancers.

6.3 Carcinoma of the Floor of the Mouth (FOM)

– The mylohyoid and hyoglossus muscles provide the muscular support for the FOM.
– Third most common site for cancer of the oral cavity.

Symptoms

Early: asymptomatic.
Late: invasion of the mandible, the root of tongue, the lingual n., the mental nerve.

Obstruction of orifice of submandibular SG resulting in its distension.

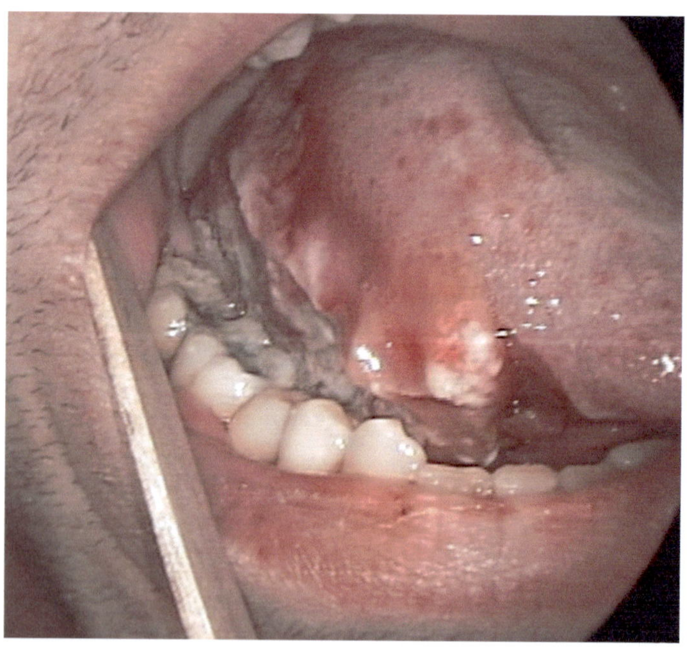

Metastases

– Cervical metastasis is most frequently seen in the submandibular (IB), upper jugular (II) and submental LN (IA).

Therapy

– Similar to that described for oral tongue cancer.

6.4   Carcinoma of the Soft Palate

– Most frequently on the oral surface of the soft palate.
– Increased incidence of additional primary tumors (13%)

Symptoms

- Early: leukoplakia, erythroplakia, or raised lesion.
- Late: Extension to tonsil, hard palate, nasopharynx.

Metastases

- Lymphatic metastases
    – up to 50% clinically present metastases at the time of
      presentation.
    – tumor thickness (>3 mm) has correlated with regional
      metastasis and survival.
    – even small midline lesions the propensity for regional
      metastasis is great (40%)
    – rate of bilateral cervical metastases: 5–15%
    – lymphatic drainage is to the upper jugular LN (II)

Therapy

– Small lesions: surgically by transoral approach, or by radia-
  tion therapy, or with the use of robotic devices.
– Larger lesions: radiation or chemoradiation.
– Because of the increased risk for bilateral LN metastases,
  treatment of both neck with ND or radiation.
– Reconstruction is difficult

6.5   Carcinoma of Tonsils

– Most common ca of the oropharynx.

Symptoms

- Early: asymptomatic
- Late: dysphagia, odynophagia, otalgia, neck mass, trismus.
- Anatomic sites of direct invasion: soft palate, tongue base, mandible, pterygoid muscles.
- Lymphatic metastases
    - Drainage to levels II–IV and retropharyngeal LN.
    - Clinically positive lymphadenopathy ranges from 66 to 76%.
    - Rate of contralateral LN meta 22%.

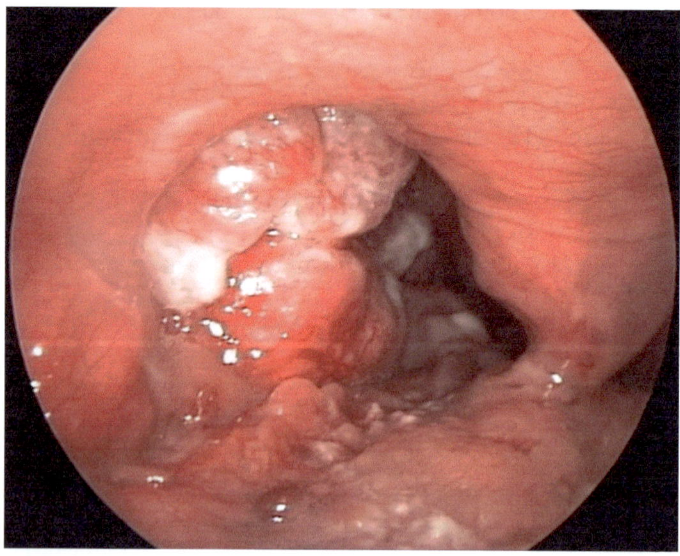

Therapy

Radiation or combined chemoradiation is the treatment of choice.

Surgical resection is useful for salvage or for patients with extensive bony invasion (approaches: transoral, anterior mandibulotomy with mandibular swing, composite resection)

Neck dissection

- before radiation or chemo-radiation in patients with N1–N3.
- posttreatment for patients with N2 or greater disease or clinically detectable disease.

Reconstructive options

- primary closure or healing by secondary intention for very small defects.
- regional pedicled flaps (pectoralis major)
- free tissue transfer (radial forearm)

6.6   Carcinoma of the Base of Tongue

- Less common and more aggressive than cancer of the oral tongue.
- Types: SCC or lymphoma.

Symptoms

- Odynophagia and referred otalgia.

Diagnosis

- Visualization of the tongue base is difficult.
- Palpation of tongue is an important part of clinical evaluation.

Metastases

- Anatomic sites of direct invasion: larynx, tonsil, soft palate and hypo-pharynx.
- Lymphatic metastases
  - More than 60% of patients have clinically detectable cervical LN meta at the time of presentation.

- Rate of bilateral cervical LN metastases: 20%
- Neck zones II–IV are the most common site for LN metastases.

Therapy

- Primarily radiation or chemoradiation.
- Surgery is used for small primary tumors or for salvage following radiation or chemoradiation.
- Surgical approaches
  1. Mandibular swing or composite resection.
  2. Median mandibulo-glossotomy (to access small tumors isolated to the mid-portion of tongue base).
  3. Suprahyoid pharyngotomy
  4. Transoral laser resection
- Laryngectomy may be necessary to prevent chronic aspiration
- Reconstruction: for total glossectomy defects a flap with significant bulk is useful (pectoralis major, rectus abdominus).

6.7   Carcinoma of Hypopharynx

<u>Hypopharynx</u> <u>subsites</u>

1. Pyriform sinus
2. Posterior hypo-pharyngeal wall
3. Postcricoid region

<u>Types</u>: Greater than 90% SCC
<u>Risk factors</u>: tobacco, alcohol, GORD, Plummer-Vinson syndrome.
<u>Site</u>: USA: pyriform sinus, EU: postcricoid

Symptoms

Early: asymptomatic
Late: Odynophagia, referred otalgia, dysphagia, hoarseness, neck mass (60–75% have palpable cervical metastases at presentation).

- Lesions that involve more than one subsite have significant increase in mortality.

Metastases

- Carcinoma of the medial pyriform wall may extend to the
  larynx.
- Posterior cricoid cancer may invade into the cricoarytenoid muscles and cartilage of the larynx.
- Lateral hypopharyngeal ca may extend to oropharynx,
  rhino-pharynx, esophagus, or prevertebral fascia.
- Tendency for sub-mucosal spread which must be taken
  into consideration during resection in order to obtain a
  negative margin.

Therapy

Treatment selection depends on stage, subsite and perfor-
mance status of the patient.

A. Radiation therapy
   • Primary modality for T1 and selected T2.
   • ND prior to radiation in certain patients with extensive
     but resectable cervical metastases.
B. Postoperative adjuvant radiation plays a crucial role fol-
   lowing surgery for advanced stage carcinomas.
   • Indications: multiple levels or bulky nodal disease, car-
     tilage invasion, ECS, positive surgical margins.
C. Concurrent chemo and RT: its roloe remains unclear.
D. Surgery
   • posterior wall: selected lesions if there is no fixation to
     prevertebral fascia, via transhyoid or median labio-
     mandibular glossotomy.
   • postcricoid: usually present at an advanced stage and
     require total laryngopharyngectomy.
   • pyriform sinus: selected T1 and T2 → extended partial
     laryngopharyngectomy. Supracricoid hemilaryngo-
     pharyngectomy (preserves cricoids and the contralateral
     arytenoids and vocal cord. Total laryngopharyngectomy
     is often required.

- transsoral endoscopic laser resection: proposed by Steiner. Elective or therapeutic ND is also performed. Surgery is followed by postoperative RT.

E. Reconstructive options
- primary closure: in selected patients with adequate mucosa.
- regional flap reconstruction: pectoralis major for partial laryngopharyngectomy. Tubed pectoralis major for total LPectomy.
- microvascular free tissue transfer: radial forearm and rectus abdominis flaps for patial pharyngectomy defects. Tubed radial forearm, rectus for closure of total LPectomy defects.
  Free jejunal autograft for total LPectomy
  Gastric pull-up when total LPectomy with esophagectomy is performed.

6.8   Nasopharyngeal Carcinoma

- Incidence: central Europe 1:100,000,
  China, South Asia and Middle East: up to 20 (consumption of salted fish containing nitrosamines and smoke from openfires).
- Predilection for middle-aged patients.
- Histology: Roughly 50% keratinizing (WHO type 1) and non-keratinizing (WHO type 2) SCC and 50% undifferentiated (WHO type 3—lymphoepithelial).
- Infection with EBV is typical for lympho-epithelial carcinoma.
- A genetic predisposition (HLA class I genotypes) is also discussed as the cause of the disease in view of its raised familial incidence.

Symptoms

- LN metastases, (usually level II or V) (the first clinical sign in 50% of cases).
  - Spread to parotid LN or retropharyngeal LN may occur.

- Serous middle ear effusion → CHL.
- Obstructed nasal air passage.
- Recurrent nose bleeding.
- Hyposmia, anosmia.

Complications

- Skull base invasion with involvement of the cranial nerves (esp. CN III–VI).
- Orbital invasion with bulbar protrusion, diplopia or ophthalmoplegia.
- Infiltration of the infratemporal fossa.
- Severe nose bleeding.
- Therapy-resistant headache.

Diagnosis

- Endoscopy: nose, nasopharynx
- Ear microscopy: retraction of TM, middle ear effusion
- Palpation: cervical lymph nodes, especially nuchal
- Inspection: mouth breathing, protrusion of the eyeball, CN deficits
- Test of cranial nerve function: especially the abducens, oculomotor, trigeminal nerve
- U/S: neck (imaging of LN in front of and behind the SCM muscle as well as nuchally).
- CT of skull and neck: to assess the extent of the tumour/ skull base ivasion.
- MRI: to assess perineural invasion and to demonstrate potential retropharyngeal LN involvement.
- Serology: Determination of serum antibodies to EBV (virus capside antigen-IgG and antigen-IgA, early antigen, nuclear antigens). Raised titres are definitive tumour markers in undifferentiated carcinomas. The titre is important for diagnosis, whereas the time course of the titre levels during and after treatment is crucial in predicting the prognosis.
- Biopsy of the naso-pharyngeal tumour in the absence of putative juvenile angiofibroma. An enlarged LN must be totally removed for histological investigation.

Additional

- PET-CT: to rule out distant metastases or to detect recurrent cancer.
- CT thorax (to rule out distant metastases).
- Ultrasound: abdomen

Therapy
Conservative treatment

- The treatment of choice

Is primary irradiation of the tumor and LN metastases with additional chemotherapy.

Surgical treatment

- They are not operated on, since radical resection is not possible. Partial resection does not improve the prognosis.
- Neck dissection (salvage surgery) is indicated in persistent cervical LN metastases after radiotherapy/chemo-radiotherapy or in recurrences in cervical LN.
- Otitis media with effusion: myringotomy with or without grommets.

Differential Diagnosis

- Craniopharyngeoma
- Juvenile angiofibroma
- Hyperplasia of the pharyngeal tonsil
- Tornwaldt's cyst

Prognosis

- In undifferentiated (lymphoepithelial) nasopharyngeal-carcinoma, the 5-year survival is about 60% for stages I and II, and about 20% for higher stages.
- In keratinizing and non-keratinizing squamous cellcarcinomas, the 5-year survival is 20%.

6.9   Carcinoma of Esophagus

- >90% of esophageal cancer is SCC or adenocarcinoma.
- >75% of ADCs occur in distal esophagus.
- SCC is more evenly distributed.
- The most common site is the lower third, followed by the middle third and rarely the cervical esophagus.
- Ca involving the cervical Es is most commonly result from extension of hypopharyngeal ca.

<u>Risk factors</u>:

SCC: tobacco, alcohol, achalasia, caustic injury, Plummer-Vinson s., history of head and neck ca, history of radiation.
ADC: Barrett's esophagus, acid reflux, tobacco, RT
Barrett's esophagus: metaplasia of the normal squamous mucosa of the distal esophagus to columnar epithelium.
Metaplastic epithelium may progress to ADC.

Symptoms

- Dysphagia
- Odynophagia
- Weight loss
- Hoarseness (if there is recurrent laryngeal n. invasion)

Metastases

- Cancer involving the cervical Es may extend to larynx and trachea (tracheo-esophageal fistula).
- Distal esophageal cancer may involve esophagogastric junction.
    - At the time of diagnosis more than 50% of patients have metastases or an unresectable primary tumor.

Diagnosis

- Barium esophagogram.
- CT scan with contrast of neck, chest, abdomen and pelvis.

- PET scan: to assess regional lymphadenopathy and detect distant meta.
- Flexible or rigid endoscopy: to assess extent and location of the lesion, obtain tissue for histopathologic diagnosis.

Therapy

A. Surgical resection
   - early stage disease is treated with a transthoracic or transhiatal approach for partial or total esophagectomy.
   - transcervical approach for upper cervical Es.
   - laryngectomy may be necessary for cervical esophageal Ca.
   - endoscopically placed stents (palliative treatment in advanced-stage disease)
B. Radiation therapy
   - primary RT used as an alternative treatment
   - postoperative RT → improves local disease control, useful on patients at high risk of recurrence, presence of residual disease
C. Chemotherapy
   - preoperative: reduction in primary tumor size and treatment of meta. NO survival benefit.
   - postoperative: the same
D. Combined chemoradiation
   - useful as primary treatment in patients with unresectable tumors.
   - preoperative: reduction in tumor size, NO survival benefit.
E. Reconstructive options.
   - Gastric transposition (pull-up) in patients undergoing total esophagectomy.
   - Cervical esophagectomy or total LPectomy is repaired with free tissue transfer: free jejuna flap, tubed radial forearm free flap, tubed pectoralis major flap.

6.10   Carcinoma of Unknown Primary (CUP) Syndrome

A biopsy-proven metastatic cancer in the absence of detectable primary tumor after an adequate diagnostic evaluation.

Symptoms

– Usually, there are no symptoms or pain
– Only aesthetic alteration caused by swollen lymph nodes.

Diagnostic Work-Up (in persistent indolent swelling of neck lymph nodes)

<u>First step</u>

- Inspection: Skin of the head/scalp
- Palpation: thyroid gland, salivary glands, tonsils, base of tongue
- Endoscopy: of pharynx and larynx, with special attention to the fossa of Rosenmüller, tonsillar region and pyriform sinuses
- Ultrasound: Floor of mouth, Neck, Thyroid gland, Parotid glands
- Audiogram/tympanogram: to exclude malfunction of Eustachian tubes (e.g. caused by an infiltrating nasopharyngeal tumour)
- FNA

<u>Second step</u>

- Biopsy

<u>Third step</u>

- MRI, CT: Head, Neck, Thorax, Abdomen/Whole-body CT
- Panendoscopy
- Bilateral submucosal biopsy from the fossae of Rosenmüller
- Bilateral tonsillectomy
- Bilateral biopsy from the base of the tongue

<u>Fourth step</u>

- PET-CT

Therapy

- In undifferentiated/anaplastic or lymphoepithelial carcinoma with positive EBV serology but without confirmed primary tumour in the nasopharynx
    - Radiotherapy of the nasopharynx and both necksides
    - Some centres recommend neck dissection, which is then followed by radiotherapy of thenasopharynx and the neck.
- Other metastases of the neck in cases with negative EBV serology, but occult primary tumour
    - Modified radical neck dissection, which is followed by radiotherapy of the affected neck side

<u>Close clinical follow-up</u>

- endoscopy, every 1–3 months
- Imaging studies (MRI or PET-CT) every 6–12 months
- Neck dissection
- Local radiotherapy, nasopharynxincluded if EBV VCA IgG/IgA, EApositive

6.11   Neck Dissection (ND)

A systematic removal of lymph nodes in the neck.

<u>Radical ND</u>: Removal of all lymph nodes from levels I to V. In addition, removal of non-lymphatic structures including the (1) spinal accessory nerve (CN XI), (2) the sternocleidomastoid muscle (SCM) and (3) the internal jugular vein (IJV) is carried out.

In patients with extensive cervical lymph node metastasis and/or extension beyond the capsule with invasion into the spinal accessory nerve, IJV, and SCM.

<u>Modified radical ND</u>: One, two or all the non-lymphatic structures (CN XI, IJV, SCM) are saved.

Type I: CN XI preserved

Type II: CN XI, IJV preserved

Type III or functional: CN XI, IJV, and SCM preserved

In patients with gross nodal metastasis to the neck that does not directly infiltrate or adhere to one, two or three of the non-lymphatic structures.

<u>Selective ND I–III (supraomohyoid ND)</u>: Removal of cervical lymph node groups I–III.

In patients with primary tumors arising from the oral cavity without clinical or radiologic evidence of cervical metastasis but who have a high probability of occult lymphatic disease.

<u>Selective neck dissection I–IV (anterolateral)</u>: Removal of cervical LN groups I–IV.

Used in treatment of oral cavity cancer patients, when metastatic disease extends to the lower part of the jugular chain.

<u>Selective ND II–IV (lateral)</u>: Removal of the jugular lymph nodes including Levels II–IV.

Used in treatment of oropharyngeal, hypopharyngeal and laryngeal cancer.

<u>Selective ND II–V (posterolateral)</u>: Excision of lymph nodes in Levels II–V and additional nodes in the suboccipital and postauricular regions.

Used to treat the neck in patients with cutaneous malignancies.

<u>Selective ND VI (dissection of the anterior compartment)</u>: Removal of LNs in Level VI.

Used in the treatment of thyroid carcinoma.

6.12   Classification of Neck Zones

Groups		Site of primary
IA Submental	LN within the triangular boundary of the anterior belly of the digastric muscles and the hyoid bone	Floor of mouth, anterior oral tongue, anterior mandibular alveolar ridge and lower lip
IB Submandibular	LN within the boundaries of the anterior and posterior bellies of the digastric muscle, the stylohyoid muscle and the body of the mandible. It includes the pre- and postglandular nodes, and the pre- and postvascular nodes	Oral cavity, anterior nasal cavity, and soft tissue structures of the mid-face, and submandibular gland
IIA Upper jugular	LN extending from the level of the skull base (above) to the level of the inferior border of the hyoid bone (below). The anterior (medial) boundary is the lateral border of the sternohyoid muscle and the stylohyoid muscle, and the posterior (lateral) boundary is the posterior border of the sternocleidomastoid muscle. Sublevel IIA nodes are located anterior (medial) to the vertical plane defined by the spinal accessory nerve	Oral cavity, nasal cavity, nasopharynx, oropharynx, hypopharynx, larynx and parotid gland

Groups		Site of primary
IIB Upper jugular	Sublevel IIB nodes are located posterior (lateral) to the vertical plane defined by the spinal accessory nerve	
III Middle jugular	LN located around the middle third of the internal jugular vein extending from the inferior border of the hyoid bone (above) to the inferior border of the cricoid cartilage (below). The anterior (medial) boundary is the lateral border of the sternohyoid muscle, and the posterior (lateral) boundary is the posterior border of the sternocleidomastoid muscle	Oral cavity, nasopharynx, oropharynx, hypopharynx, and larynx
IV Lower jugular	LN located around the lower third of the IJV extending from the inferior border of the cricoid (above) to the clavicle (below). The anterior (medial) boundary is the lateral border of the sternohyoid muscle, and the posterior (lateral) boundary is the posterior border of the sternocleidomastoid muscle	Hypopharynx, cervical esophagus, and larynx

(continued)

Groups		Site of primary
VA and VB Posterior triangle	LNs located along the lower half of the spinal accessory nerve and the transverse cervical artery, along with the supraclavicular nodes. The superior boundary is the apex formed by a convergence of the SCM and the trapezius muscles, the inferior boundary is the clavicle, the anterior (medial) boundary is the posterior border of the sternocleidomastoid muscle, and the posterior (lateral) boundary is the anterior border of the trapezius muscle. Sublevel VA is separated from Sublevel VB by a horizontal plane marking the inferior border of the arch of the cricoid cartilage. Sublevel VA includes the spinal accessory nodes	Nasopharynx and oropharynx (sublevel VA), and the thyroid gland (sublevel VB)
VB Posterior triangle	Sublevel VB includes the nodes following the transverse cervical vessels and the supraclavicular nodes. (Virchow's node is located in level IV).	

Groups		Site of primary
VI Anterior (central) compartment	LN in this compartment include the pre- and paratracheal nodes, the precricoid (Delphian) node, and the perithyroidal nodes, including the LNs along the recurrent laryngeal nerves. The superior boundary is the hyoid bone, the inferior boundary is the suprasternal notch, and the lateral boundaries are the common carotid arteries	Thyroid gland, glottic and subglottic larynx, apex of the pyriform sinus, and cervical esophagus

Cutaneous Neoplasms

6.13 Basal Cell Carcinoma

– The most common skin cancer.
  <u>Risk factors</u>: sun exposure, older age, fair skin
  It spreads by direct local invasion.
  It does not have metastatic behavior.

Symptoms

– Erythematous lesion with raised margins.

Diagnosis

– Biopsy

Therapy

– Wide local excision.

6.14   Squamous Cell Carcinoma

- The second most common cutaneous carcinoma.
- It frequently affects elderly people with a phenotype of red hair, blue eyes and fair skin, who for a long time have been chronically exposed to UV.

Symptoms

- The lesion presents as a painless plaque-like or verrucous tumor that can ultimately progress to being large, necrotic, and infected.

Diagnosis

- Biopsy

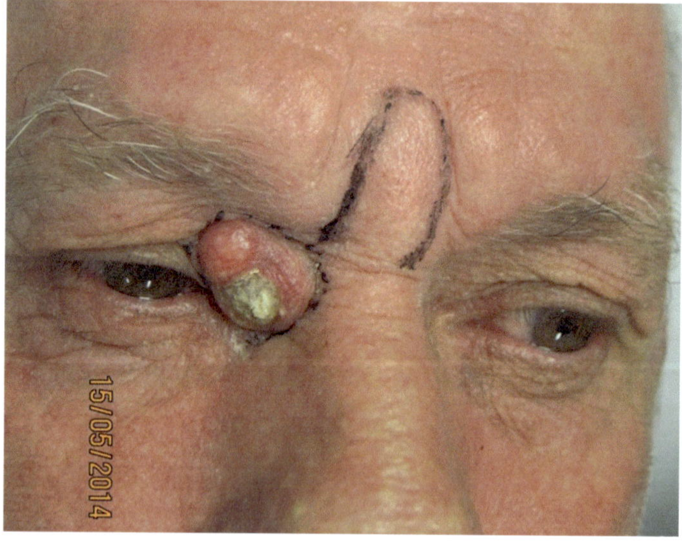

Therapy

- Wide surgical excision: not as effective as surgery in conjunction with radiation therapy.
- Radiotherapy: it has some success as a monotherapy in low-risk or cosmetically sensitive areas such as the external ear, eyelid or nose.

6.15   Melanoma

<u>Risk factors</u>

- Sun exposure [ultraviolet (UV) light causes a photo-chemical reaction in DNA].
- Tanning beds
- Fair skin, blond or red hair
- Family history of melanoma
- Freckling of the upper back.

Diagnosis

- History and Physical examination
    - Common characteristics of melanoma (ABCDE checklist):
      Assymetry, Border irregularities, Color variegation, Diameter >6 mm or recent increase in size, Evolution (changes in size, color)
    - Location has a significant impact on prognosis: head and neck melanoma has a worse prognosis than other sites.
    - Signs of aggressive disease: (1) ulceration, (2) nodurality, (3) satellite lesions
    - Thorough examination of the draining LN basin is required.
- Imaging
    - Chest X-ray: Stage I or II unless suspicion for distant metastases exists
    - CT with contrast of the head and neck: to evaluate the extent of local-regional disease.
    - Metastatic imaging workup includes:
      A. CT of chest, abdomen and pelvis with contrast
      B. MRI of brain
      C. Recently, PET
    - Metastatic evaluation is required in:
      (a) Patients with thick melanomas (>4 mm), satellitosis, ulceration or recurrent lesions.
      (b) Patients with regional metastases (stage III)
      (c) Patients with signs of metastatic disease on examination or laboratory evaluation.
      (d) Patients with known systemic disease (stage IV).

- Biopsy
- Excisional biopsy
  - A. Acceptable if lesion is very small
  - B. Excise with 1–2 mm margins (wide excision necessary if pathologic review yields melanoma).
  - C. May disrupt lymphatic drainage
- Incisional biopsy
  - A. Allows adequate assessment of depth of invasion.
  - B. Does not disrupt border of tumor (in order to determine appropriate margins for wide local excision).
  - C. Does not affect lymphatic drainage (if lymphoscintigraphy is planned).
- Staging
- Most important prognostic factors: depth of invasion, ulceration, mitotic index, satellitosis, degree of LN involvement and distant meta.

Therapy
Surgery

A. <u>Primary lesion</u>

- Wide local excision (unless systemic metastases are present and palliative resection is unwarranted).
- Margins:
  1. 1 cm for tumors of <1 mm thick
  2. >1 cm for 1–2 mm
  3. 2 cm for >2 mm thick.

B. <u>Cervical lymph nodes</u>

- Therapeutic ND
  - Evidence of lymphatic metastasis
  - Anterior scalp, temple, ear or facial melanomas require superficial parotidectomy as well
  - Posterior scalp, ear melanomas require postauricular and sub-occipital LN removal.
- Elective ND
  - Has been largely replaced by SLNB
  - Evaluation of draining lymphatics in patients with T2 or T3 tumors and N0 neck.

- Also for lesions extending to Clark levels IV or V, lesions with an increased mitotic index, or ulceration
- Parotid LN and neck levels IB, II, III, and IV are at risk when lesion involve the anterior scalp, temple, facial lesions and ear.
- Posterior scalp and retro-auricular lesions drain to levels II, III, IV and V, along with the retroauricular and suboccipital LN.
- Sentinel LN biopsy (SLNB)
  - SLNs positive for metastatic melanoma necessitates complete ND

Conservative treatment

- External beam radiation
  - It is used in three settings:
    1. Postoperative following ND of palpable lymphatic disease.
    2. RT to regional LN from patients with T2b to T4, N0 disease, who cannot undergone SLNB or ND
    3. Regional recurrence after ND.

- Chemotherapy
  - It is used in two settings:
    1. patients with distant metastases.
    2. patients at high risk for distant metastases

6.16   Merkel Cell Carcinoma

An aggressive neuroendocrine carcinoma arising in the dermoepidermal junction.

- It occurs most frequently in sun-exposed areas of skin, particularly the head and neck, followed by the extremities, and then the trunk

- It typically affects fair-skinned individuals over the age of 50.
- While MCC is 30 times rarer than melanoma, it is twice as lethal

Symptoms

- It appears as a painless, indurated, solitary dermal nodule and rarely as an ulcer.
- These tumors are typically red, blue or skin-colored and vary greatly in size.
- At the time of presentation, MCC tumors are often considered benign by patients and physicians alike.
- It is common for MCC to have spread to lymph nodes at the time of diagnosis even though the nodes are not enlarged or detectable on physical examination. Even a small MCC has a 30% chance of having spread to LN by the time of diagnosis.

Diagnosis

- Computed tomography (CT) scan of the chest and abdomen to rule out primary small cell lung cancer as well as distant and regional metastases.
- Sentinel lymph node biopsy (SLNB): to determine whether the MCC has spread to the lymph nodes and is a very important in a patient's prognosis.

Therapy

- Wide local excision to reduce the risk of local recurrence
- Radiation therapy: because of apparent radiosensitivity of MCC, and the high incidence of local and regional recurrences.
- Chemotherapy.

Further Readings

1. Koivunen P, Bäck L, Laranne J, Irjala H. Unknownprimary: diagnostic issues in the biological endoscopy and positron emission tomography scan era. Curr Opin Otolaryngol Head Neck Surg. 2015;23(2):121–6.
2. Brummer GC, Bowen AR, Bowen GM. Merkel cell carcinoma: current issues regarding diagnosis, management, and emerging treatment strategies. Am J Clin Dermatol. 2016;17(1):49–62.

Chapter 7
Oesophagus

7.1 Pharyngo-Oesophageal Diverticula (Zenker Diverticulum)

Protrusion of posterior hypopharyngeal mucosa between the oblique and transverse fibres of cricopharyngeal muscle (Killian's triangle).

Symptoms

Dysphagia/odynophagia, globe/foreign body feeling, regurgitation of undigested food, fetor ex ore, and aspiration (recurring pneumonitis).

Diagnosis

- Barium swallow: demonstrates a fluid filled sac.
- Endoscopy is quite hazardous because the sac has no muscular component and is easily perforated.

Therapy

1. Conventional excision (diverticulectomy) or diverticulopexy through a left-sided cervicotomy combined with a long myotomy of the cricopharyngeal muscle.

P. Koltsidopoulos et al., *ENT*,
DOI 10.1007/978-3-319-56330-5_7,
© Springer International Publishing AG 2017

2. Endoscopic division of the cricopharyngeal bar with CO_2 Laser (the mucosal surface of the diverticulum should be examined endocopically to rule out SCC).
3. Endocopic division with a stapler (Endo-GIA-30)

7.2   Gastro-Oesophageal Reflux Disease

> Any condition in which symptoms or histo-pathologic changes result from refluxed gastric acid.

- GORD affects 7–10% of the population on a daily basis, and 40% on a monthly basis.
- A certain amount of acid reflux is normal and occurs after meal. Whether it becomes pathologic depends on: frequency, volume, duration of exposure

Defence mechanisms against GORD are:

- A competent lower oesophageal sphincter
- Peristaltic clearance of oesophageal acid
- Oesophageal epithelial resistance
- A competent upper oesophageal sphincter
  - Although the pH of the refluxate is important, it is pepsin concentration that seems to be responsible for the mucosal injury.

Symptoms

- The most common symptom of GORD is heartburn, a retro-sternal and epigastric pain that may radiate to the back, arm, pharynx and ear.
- Occasionally it must be distinguished from cardiac pain (if it dissipates rapidly with nitroglycerine, it is unlikely to be oesophageal in origin).

<u>Oesophageal Symptoms</u>

- Heartburn
- Regurgitation
- Dysphagia
- Chest pain.

<u>Extraoesophageal Syndromes</u>

- Pharyngitis
- Laryngitis
- Chronic cough
- Asthma
- Sinusitis
- Recurrent otitis media

Therapy

A. When symptoms of GORD are typical and the patient responds to therapy, no diagnostic tests are necessary.
B. If the patient fails to respond or has atypical symptoms, a number of tests are available:
   - The 24-h pH probe is the definite test for reflux.
   - Endoscopy may show characteristic mucosa changes in the distal oesophagus. However, the presence of normal-appearing mucosa does not rule out the possibility of reflux disease (50% of patients with symptomatic reflux have normal findings on endoscopy).
   - ENT examination (posterior laryngitis, granuloma of the vocal cord) to detect extraoesophageal syndromes.
   - Dietary changes [avoiding foods that are acidic (citrus fruits) or foods that can cause gastric reflux (fatty or fried foods, coffee or tea)].
   - Lifestyle changes (smoking cessation, weight reduction, avoidance of eating within 3 h before bedtime.
   - Medical therapy: Proton pump inhibitors (for 8–12 weeks).
   - Surgical therapy: Only when medical therapy fails, the so-called antireflux surgery is indicated.

7.3   Caustic Ingestion

- In children, in mentally retarded adults and in adults trying to commit suicide.
- The most common agents are alkaline (60%) (e.g. sodium or potassium hydroxides, found in many household cleaners, and acid corrosives).

<u>Pathophysiology</u>

- Alkalis tend to penetrate faster than acids, causing a liquefaction necrosis that may extend rapidly through the mucosa to the underlying muscle of the oesophagus.
- Acids produce a coagulation necrosis with superficial eschar that helps to prevent deeper penetration.
- Liquid products are more easily swallowed and produce the most damage at normal narrowings within the oesophagus.
- Solid substances may attach to the oral mucosa and are more difficult to swallow, thereby more often causing damage to the oral cavity and pharynx.

Symptoms

- Burning of the lips, tongue or pharynx and dysphagia.
- Excessive salivation with drooling
- If airway is involved: wheezing and stridor
- If oesophageal perforation occurs: severe chest pain, subcutaneous emphysema, sepsis and shock may
- If gastric injury occurs: haematemesis and abdominal pain

Diagnosis

1. Typical history (accidental or suicidal ingestion)
2. Typical clinical findings.
3. Radiographic evaluation (X-ray of chest and abdomen). A more sensitive study is CT of the chest.
4. Flexible endoscopy: to assess the extent of injury. It should be done within the first 48–72 h. After this time, the risk of perforation during the endoscopy is much higher. The examination is most safely done with a paediatric endoscope with

minimal air insufflation. When the first injury is recognized, further endoscopy has to be done with extreme caution to avoid mucosal injury, creating a false lumen and full-thickness perforation.

Therapy

- Goal: preventing of oesophageal stricture or perforation.
- Acute measures: airway management and volume substitution
- Prompt administration of broad-spectrum antibiotics (they decrease the bacterial load and the formation of granulation tissue, they prevent intramural spread and possibly mediastinitis) and steroids.
- Steroids: their use is controversial.
- Early dilatation is useful and necessary in stricture formation. It should be started in the fifth or sixth week after injury. The incidence and interval of repeated dilatations depends on the degree of stenosis.
- The early placement of a nasogastric tube has been advocated by some groups to prevent stenosis.

Late Risks

- Up to 13% of patients with a caustic injury will develop a SCC, even years or decades after injury. Therefore, regular endoscopic control is necessary.

7.4   Oesophageal Perforation

Etiology:

- Iatrogenic (the most common cause)
- External Trauma
- Spontaneous Rupture

Iatrogenic Perforation

- Sites of involvement: the cervical oesophagus at the cricopharyngeus and the thoracoabdominal oesophagus at the diaphragmatic hiatus.

- Associated procedures: endoscopic manipulation or dilatation, placement of a nasogastric tube, traumatic endotracheal intubation or dilatative tracheotomy.
  - Injury at the crico-pharyngeus (USO) happens because of:
    1. Introduction of the oesophagoscope into the pyriform sinus
    2. Narrowing of UOS
    3. Prominent cervical osteophytes
- Injury at diaphragmatic hiatus tends to occur as the oesophagus angles anteriorly towards the diaphragm, which is often not appreciated by the endoscopist.

<u>External Trauma</u>

- Penetrating trauma
- Sudden high pressure (blunt trauma)

<u>Spontaneous Rupture (Boerhaave syndrome)</u>

- It is caused by severe vomiting.
- The majority of spontaneous perforations occur in the distaloesophagus, where it seems to be an inherent weakness within the left posterolateral wall.

Symptoms
Perforation of the cervical oesophagus:

- Neck pain (more than 90%)
- Subcutaneous emphysema (more than 50%)
- Dysphagia and odynophagia
- Fever and leucocytosis will develop over the first 24 h.

Distal perforation:

- Retrosternal chest pain or shoulder pain
- Problems and pain with respiration
- Subcutaneous emphysema

Diagnosis

- It is extremely important to make the diagnosis rapidly. Delays in diagnosis and treatment are associated with increased mortality.

- History
  - Persistent pain and fever after oesophagoscopy should alert the clinician.
  - Note that 50% of patients will be asymptomatic for the first 8 h after injury.

- Radiology
  - A water-soluble contrast medium, such as Gastrografin, is used for the oesophagogram and confirms perforation in about 80% of cases. Gastrografin is preferable because it causes less mediastinal inflammation. However, if the test is negative, a thin-barium swallow may demonstrate the perforation because it remains more sensitive.
  - Lateral cervical radiographs: show widening of the retrooesophageal space and streaks of air in the soft tissue planes (prevertebral air) and subcutaneous or cervical emphysema.
  - Chest radiographs: may demonstrate pneumomediastinum, mediastinal widening or pneumothorax
  - CT with contrast: helpful if an abscess is suspected.

Therapy

- Therapy should begin even before the perforation has been verified.
- Controversy as to whether medical therapy alone is adequate or whether all oesophageal perforations need surgical intervention.

- <u>Perforation of the cervical oesophagus</u>:
  - i.v. high-dose antibiotics (clindamycin, ampicillin, sulbactam).
  - i.v. hydration and alimentation (allowing nothing per mouth).
  - Nasogastric suction (for nutritional support) if the tube can be safely passed.
  - Close monitoring. Any deterioration in overall status or signs of sepsis will necessitate surgical drainage.

- In cervical perforation there is a clear trend to medical therapy alone. Appropriate treatment depends on the site and size of the perforation, the time since the injury happened and the health status of the patient.

- <u>Perforation of middle and lower oesophagus</u>
  - There is a higher complication rate
  - A combined surgical and medical therapy is usually favoured.

7.5   Foreign Bodies

- Oesophagus is the most common site of foreign body impaction within the gastrointestinal tract.

Adults: history of having eaten fish or chicken.
Children: the history may be very misleading.

Symptoms

- Dysphagia
- Odynophagia
- Drooling.

Diagnosis

- Radiographs: both antero-posterior and lateral neck films and a chest X-ray.
- Negative X-ray findings do not rule out a foreign body.
  - In case of clinically or radiologically suspected foreign body, endoscopy is necessary.
  - Foreign body endoscopy is an ENT emergency.

Therapy

- Endoscopy in the first 6 h with a rigid oesophagoscope and removal of the foreign body.
  If disk battery is ingested, it should be emergently removed (it may release a caustic solution and cause injury to the mucosa).

- After removal, patients need to be observed for any signs of perforation.
  A Gastografin contrast study is done before oral food intake is resumed.

Further Readings

1. Johnson CM, Postma GN. Zenker diverticulum—which surgical approach is superior? JAMA Otolaryngol Head Neck Surg. 2016;142(4):401–3.
2. Park KS. Evaluation and management of caustic injuries from ingestion of acid or alkaline substances. Clin Endosc. 2014;47(4):301–7.
3. Leinwand K, Brumbaugh DE, Kramer RE. Button battery ingestion in children: a paradigm for management of severe pediatric foreign body ingestions. Gastrointest Endosc Clin N Am. 2016;26(1):99–118.

Chapter 8
Rhinopharynx

8.1 Adenoid Hypertrophy

A common disease of the childhood characterized by hyperplasia of the adenoids owing to chronic inflammation or allergy of the upper airway.

Causative organisms: Streptococcus pneumonia, Haemophilus influenza

– Almost exclusively in children.

Symptoms

- Nasal obstruction
- Mouth breathing
- Hyponasality (rhinophonia clausa)
- Sleep disorders: snoring, obstructive sleep apnoea syndrome
- Recurrent mucopurulent rhinorrhoea
- Conductive HL
- Lack of appetite owing to reduced ability to smell
- Delay in development

P. Koltsidopoulos et al., *ENT*,
DOI 10.1007/978-3-319-56330-5_8,
© Springer International Publishing AG 2017

Complications

- Recurrent purulent rhinopharyngitis.
- Congestive sinusitis, sinubronchial syndrome.
- Otitis media with effusion.
- Recurrent AOM.
- Development of a gothic palate.
- Malocclusion of teeth.
- Dental caries.

Diagnosis

- Inspection: adenoid facies (narrow, pale, dumb facial expression with open mouth and sunken eyes), driedmucus in the nasal orifice (external nares), eczema of the nasal orifice, sometimes halitosis
- Palpation: cervical lymph nodes, also nuchal
- Inspection and if possible endoscopy of nasal cavities, buccal cavity, oro-pharynx and nasopharynx: tooth malalignment, malocclusion, gothic palate, often also tonsillar hyperplasia, secretion at the dorsal wall of the pharynx
- Otomicroscopy: retracted TM with or without middle ear effusion
- Tympanometry and stapedius reflexes: flattympanogram, reflexes often absent
- Pure tone audiogram

Therapy

Conservative treatment: only preoperatively or when surgery is contraindicated:

- Antibiotics: amoxicillin, macrolides.
- Decongestants
- When surgery is contra-indicated, long-term treatment with corticoid nasal sprays.

Surgical treatment

- Surgical removal of the adenoids is the first-line treatment!
- Adenoidectomy: any adenoid hyperplasia with chronically obstructed nasal breathing, recurrent or persistent rhino-

genic infections, chronic purulent rhinorrhoea, congestive sinusitis, persistent or recurrent disorder of tube function, otitis media or mucotympanum, chronicbronchitis or in sleep apnoea syndrome.
- Sleep apnea syndrome: simultaneous removal of tonsils (tonsillectomy).
- Adenoidectomy is only rarely indicated in cleft-palate patients.
- Simultaneous reconstruction of the velo-pharynx may be necessary because of the danger of swallowing disturbance and hypernasality.

8.2 Tornwaldt's Cyst

A benign midline nasopharyngeal mucosal cyst.

- Irregular notochord regression in the sixth week of gestation leads to its formation

Symptoms

- Almost always asymptomatic
- If cyst becomes infected: halitosis or periodic discharge of foul tasting fluid into the mouth
- Otitis media with effusion due to obstruction of the Eustachian tube.

Diagnosis

- In most cases it is found incidentally.
- Endoscopy
- CT: well circumscribed, low density (fluid density centrally), non-enhancing lesion

Therapy

- Asymptomatic lesions require no treatment.
- If treatment is required: marsupialization of the cyst (de-roofing).

Further Reading

1. Christmas DA Jr, Yanagisawa E, Mirante JP. Endoscopic view of obstructing nasopharyngeal cysts (Tornwaldt's cysts). Ear Nose Throat J. 2007;86(10):591–2.

Chapter 9
Pharynx

9.1   Acute Streptococcal Pharyngo-Tonsillitis

A bacterial infection of the tonsils with group A β-haemolytic streptococcus, rarely with staphylococcus and haemophilus.

– Most commonly occurs in children aged 5–6 years.

Symptoms

– Odynophagia
– Fever
– Lymphadenopathy
– Dry sore throat.

Complications

Peritonsillar, retropharyngeal or parapharyngeal abscess.

Airway obstruction, deep neck infection, septicaemia, meningitis, mediastinitis and thrombophlebitis of the jugular vein.

Poststreptococcal glomerulonephritis. Acute rheumatic fever.

P. Koltsidopoulos et al., *ENT*,
DOI 10.1007/978-3-319-56330-5_9,
© Springer International Publishing AG 2017

Diagnosis

- Inspection: erythematous pharyngeal mucosa, swollen and red tonsils, with yellow spots, malodorous breath. In some cases tonsils touch each other in the midline (kissing tonsils).
- High white cell blood counts and high concentration of CRP.
- Throat culture is only necessary during a rapid or recurrent course.

Therapy

- Penicillin V for a 10-day course.
- In patients allergic to penicillin → clindamycin or erythromycin.
- Patients with recurrent tonsilar infections (6–7 per year, several episodes for two or more consecutive years) need to undergo tonsillectomy.

9.2   Complications of Oropharyngeal Infections

<u>Non-suppurative complications</u>

9.2.1   *Scarlet Fever*

- Caused by streptococci, which produce a pathognomonic erythrogenic exotoxin.
- High fever, dysphagia, a yellow membrane covering the tonsils.
- An erythematous rash beginning on thorax, spreading all over the body and excluding the perioral region.
- "Strawberry tongue" (caused by desquamation of tongue)

Therapy

- Penicillin for 10 days

9.2.2 *Acute Rheumatic Fever*

- Occurs 15–20 days after a pharyngeal infection with group A β-haemolytic streptococci.

Pathophysiology: Production of cross-reactive antibodies, which react with heart tissue, causing endocarditis, myocarditis, and pericarditis.

Therapy

Patients need therapy with penicillin or have to undergo tonsillectomy.

9.2.3 *Post-streptococcal Glomerulonephritis*

- Occurs 10 days after a pharyngotonsillar infection with group A β-haemolytic streptococcus.
- The incidence is 10–25%.

Pathophysiology: Immune complexes and circulating auto-antibodies of the streptococcal antigen damage the glomerulus, and acute nephritic syndrome occurs.

Therapy
- Patients need therapy with penicillin or have to undergo tonsillectomy.

Suppurative complications.

9.2.4 *Peritonsillary Abscess (Quinsy)*

Abscess that lies in the space between the tonsillar capsule and the surrounding pharyngeal muscle bed.

- Typical localizations are the upper pole and along the palate-glossal arch.
- The process starts with an infection of the tonsils and cellulitis of the surrounding tissues and progresses into an abscess beyond the tonsillar capsule.

- The abscess usually occurs in patients with recurrent acute tonsillitis and with chronic tonsillitis, which stays untreated. It is more common in young adults.
- Patients present with a history of acute tonsillar infection and sometimes with initial improvement, if they received medication.

Symptoms

- Symptoms intensify during development of the abscess.
- Odynophagia, sometimes with dehydration.
- Unilateral soreness,
- Drooling and
- Trismus;
- Otalgia on the affected side may occur.

Complications

- Spread into the deep neck spaces
- Septicaemia
- Mediastinitis.
- Airway obstruction

Diagnosis

- Inspection: swollen and bulging palate, displacement of the affected tonsil to the midline and deviation of the uvula to the healthy side.
- Palpation: Swollen and tender cervical LN.
- Needle aspiration may confirm the diagnosis. Microbiologic examination shows a mixed infection with aerobic and anaerobic bacteria.
- Ultrasound may verify the diagnosis.
- It can be difficult to differentiate peritonsillar cellulitis from a true abscess (the favoured option is to treat the infection initially with i.v. antibiotics and hydration. If the patients improve within 24 h, the infection is mostly cellulitis).

Therapy

Opening of the abscess by aspiration or incision and intravenous antibiotics as well as careful follow-up.
- Aminopenicillin or cephalosporin IV may be indicated.

- After treatment of the acute infection, patients should undergo tonsillectomy because of the high recurrence rate.
- Another treatment is a "quinsy tonsillectomy" (tonsillectomy during acute infection).

9.2.5   Parapharyngeal Abscess

- Parapharyngeal space starts superiorly at the skull base and ends inferiorly at the level of the hyoid bone.
- Medial boundary: superior constrictor muscle, Lateral margin: mandible, parotid and pterygoid muscle, Posterior boundary: prevertebral fascia.
- Divided into anterior and posterior division by the styloid process. The carotids and the cranial nerves are located in this space, so an abscess may spread along these structures.

Pus from the tonsillar region may go through the superior constrictor musclealong preformed openings of nerves and vessels.

Symptoms

- Odynophagia
- Drooling
- Pain of the throat and neck and tender swelling of the neck, in the region of the angle of the mandible.
- Trismus may also be present owing to inflammation and oedema around the pterygoid musculature. (If only the posterior compartment of the parapharyngeal space is involved, there may be no trismus, but rather swelling of the posterior pharyngeal wall and of the posterior pillar).

Diagnosis

- Inspection: tonsillitis, asymmetric pharyngeal swelling, if the abscess extends more inferiorly, airway obstruction may occur.
- CT scan: for definitive diagnosis.

Therapy

- Surgical drain: the safest approach to the para-pharyngeal space is through a lateral cervical approach. The great vessels need to be identified.
- Control of the airway.
- Intravenous antibiotics adapted to the disease.

9.2.6   Retro-Pharyngeal Abscess

- The retropharyngeal space lies behind the pharynx, anterior to the prevertebral fascia.
- It extends from the skull base to the tracheal bifurcation. Behind oesophagus the space is called "retrooesophageal space".
- In the space there are two layers of LN.
- The RA often occurs in children. It rarely occurs in adults; tuberculosis may be the most common diagnosis.

Symptoms

- Trismus
- Drooling
- Dyspnoea
- Dysphagia
- The anterior longitudinal ligament may be affected, so the head cannot be moved.
- Fever and malaise.

Diagnosis

- Inspection: a fluctuant mass at the posterior wall of the pharynx and oedema of the pharynx and larynx.
- X-ray and ultrasound: may show abscess formation.
- CT scan: the most important diagnostic tool. It shows a hypo-dense retropharyngeal region with a ring-form enhancement. The presence of air confirms the diagnosis.

Therapy

- Surgical drainage and i.v. antibiotics.
- A vertical incision followed by blunt dissection is made just off the midline in the posterior pharyngeal wall. Intubation may be difficult, the abscess cavity may be injured and infectious material may be aspirated.

9.2.7   Lemierre's Syndrome

It is characterized by thrombophlebitis of the internal jugular vein (IJV) and bacteremia caused by anaerobic organisms, following a recent oropharyngeal infection.

Causative agent: *Fusobacterium necrophorum*.
Pathophysiology: Bacterium passage from tonsillar vein to IJV. Bacterial endotoxin induces platelet aggregation and septic thrombus formation.
   Potential fatal complication

Symptoms

- Sore throat
- Neck mass
- Neck tenderness
- Spiking "picket fence" fevers
- Lethargy
- Septic emboli

Diagnosis

- CT with contrast: filling defect in IJV
- Tobey-Ayer test: compression of the thrombosed IJV during spinal tap does not increase CSF pressure

Therapy

- Prolonged antibiotic therapy
- Anticoagulants (the use of them is controversial)
- Surgical treatment (drainage of abscesses in the neck, IJV ligation or excision is rare).

9.3   Infectious Mononucleosis

Pathogen: **Epstein-Barr virus**.
   It is transmitted by oral contact and is also called "*kissing disease*".

– Incubation period of up to 4 weeks.

Symptoms

– Severe attack of acute tonsillitis.
– Cervical adenopathy
– Fever
– Malaise
– Hepatosplenomegaly

Diagnosis
– Inspection: severely enlarged tonsils, covered with extensive grey-white exudates.
– Blood tests:
   1. Elevated lymphocytes (atypical in structure)
   2. Epstein–Barr virus specific antibody serologic test: positive result
   3. Monospot test: positive
   4. Liver enzymes: to exclude liver affection.
– Ultrasound findings of the liver should also be obtained.

Therapy

– Supportive: bed rest, intravenous fluids, anti-inflammatory drugs and analgesia.
– Antibiotics: to avoid bacterial superinfection at the beginning of the disease, during leucocytopenia (no amoxycillin or ampicillin → generalized maculopapular exanthema).
– Patients with hepato-splenomegaly should avoid physical activity for almost 3 months.
– In case of progressive airway obstruction due to tonsillar swelling, a short course of steroids may be helpful.

9.4 Herpangina

Tonsillar infection with Coxsackie virus.

Symptoms

- Ulcerative vesicles over the tonsils, pharynx and soft palate.
- Palmar and plantar vesicles may occur (hand, foot and mouth disease).
- General symptoms such as headache, malaise, fever, odynophagia and lymphadenitis.
- Increasing concentration of antibodies against Coxsackie virus

Therapy

Symptomatic.
Antiviral medication with aciclovir may be tried.

9.5 PFAPA (Periodic Fever, Aphthous Stomatitis, Pharyngitis, Adenitis) Syndrome

It is a periodic fever syndrome that includes symptoms of pharyngitis, aphthous stomatitis, and pharyngitis, and adenitis.

- Episodes of fever start suddenly and last for 3–7 days.
- Fevers occur routinely every few weeks.
- The disease may last for several years but usually will resolve by itself in the second decade of life.
- The disease onset is generally before the age of 5 years.
- Etiology is unknown.

Symptoms

- Recurrent episodes of fever with aphthous stomatitis and pharyngitis.
- Occasionally, there also may be exudate and usually the lymph nodes in the neck are enlarged (adenitis).
- Additional features, including headache, gastrointestinal symptoms, rash, and arthralgia, may be present but are not consistently noted.

Diagnosis

- There are no laboratory tests specific for diagnosing PFAPA.
- The disease is diagnosed based on symptoms and physical examination.
- The differential diagnosis includes: Streptococcus infection, cyclic neutropenia and the hereditary periodic fever syndromes (HPFs).

Therapy

- The aim of the treatment will be to control symptoms during the episodes of fever, to shorten the duration of the episodes, and to prevent episodes from occurring.
- Use of steroids at the start of an episode can stop it, but also may shorten the time to the next episode.
- PFAPA usually resolves spontaneously during the second decade of life. Tonsillectomy may cure the disease.
- Tonsillectomy cures PFAPA in the majority of patients (more than 80%)

9.6   Vincent's Angina

<u>Pathogens</u>: Caused by Treponema vincentii and Spirochaeta denticulata (they both exist in the normal flora of mouth).
<u>Risk groups</u>: In patients with poor oral hygiene and lowered resistance.

Diagnosis
Inspection: one tonsil shows a white, necrotizing exudative membrane sometimes combined with an ulcerative lesion.

Significant is the difference between local symptoms and the good general feeling of the patient.

D/D

Acute tonsillitis, syphilis, diphtheria, neoplasm.
Unilateral pain on swallowing, fever, sore throat and cervical lymphadenopathy.

Therapy

– Antibiotics (penicillin)
– Aggressive oral hygiene

9.7   Diphteria

Pathogen: **Corynebacterium diphtheria**

Symptoms

– Sore throat, low-grade fever and cervical lymphadenopathy.
– Sometimes malaise, headache and nausea.
– Sweet fetor ex ore.

Diagnosis

– Inspection: Grey, velvety, firm adherent pseudo-membranes covering the tonsils. When the membranes are wiped, the underlying surface bleeds easily.
– Direct cultures should be obtained for smear and culture tests. It may be spread systemically and lead to myocarditis, nephritis and ancephalitis.

  D/D
  Infectious mononucleosis, candidiasis and acute pharyngitis.

Therapy

– Antitoxin should be given within the first 48 h (allergy testing against horse serum needs to be done before application).
– Antibiotics are ineffective against the circulating toxin, but symptoms in patients who are treated early with penicillin may be less severe.

– Isolation precautions: the patient needs to be isolated for 2–4 after the end of the therapy.

9.8   Lingual Tonsillar Infection

Bacterial pathogens are similar to those of acute tonsillitis. Occurs usually in adults, (especially in immune-compromised or in patients with diabetes).

Symptoms

Severe pain, sore throat, dysphagia, dyspnea.
Complication: Airway obstruction may occur if inflammation spreads to epiglottis.

Diagnosis

Red and swollen lingual tonsil with yellow spots.

Therapy

Macrolides or penicillin V for 10 days.

9.9   Lingual Cysts

In the floor of the tongue or into the vallecula.

Symptoms

– Dysphagia
– Inspection

Therapy

– Surgical excision

9.10   Chronic Tonsillitis

Recurrent infections of tonsils and of the peritonsillar tissue lead to permanent inflammation in the tonsillar crypts and scarring of the tonsillar tissue. Bacteria may grow in the badly drained crypts.

<u>Causative organisms</u>: similar to those which cause acute infection, with a predominance of β-haemolytic streptococci.

Symptoms

Recurrent or persistent sore throats, dysphagia, malaise, malodorous tonsillar concretions as well as fetor ex ore.
Cervical adenopathy.

Diagnosis

- Inspection: tonsils may be covered with debris or there may be purulent material in the tonsillar crypts. They appear atrophic and scared, often with surrounding peritonsillar erythematous tissue.
- Blood count: increased number of WBC and increased concentration of antistreptolysin.

Therapy

- Analgesics, and antibiotics when indicated.
- Tonsillectomy is generally suggested when the patient complains of recurrent infections of more than 5–7 per year or several infections in two or more subsequent years.

9.11   Sleep Apnea Syndrome

> A potentially serious sleep disorder characterized by pauses in breathing during sleep.

- **Definitions**:

  - Apneic event: cessation of ventilation for 10 s or longer leading to an arousal
  - Hypopneic event: a decrease in airflow of 30% with a 4% decrease in oxygen saturation or a 50% decrease in airflow with a 3% decrease in oxygen saturation

- Respiratory effort-related arousal (RERA): absence of apnea–hypopnea with a 10 s or more duration of progressive negative esophageal pressure leading to an arousal or microarousal
- Apnea Index (AI): number of apneas in an hour period
- Respiratory distress index (RDI): number of apneas, hypopneas

Symptoms

- Loud snoring
- Witnessed episodes of gasping or choking
- Frequent movements that disrupt sleep
- Restless sleep regardless of time slept
- Fatigue
- Excessive daytime sleepiness (Epworth score)
- Forgetfulness
- Irritability
- Sexual dysfunction
- Motor vehicle accidents
- Job-related accidents

Complications

1. Increased mortality
2. Cardiovascular disease
    - Hypertension
    - Coronary artery disease
    - Congestive heart failure
    - Arrhythmia
    - Myocardial infarcts
    - Stroke
    - Risk for insulin resistance
    - Sudden death
    - Pulmonary hypertension
3. Neurocognitive difficulties
    - Problems with attention, working memory and executive function
4. Increased risk of motor vehicle or job-related accidents

Diagnosis

- Screening
  - Epworth Sleepiness Scale Score > 10
- Rule out other disorders causing fatigue
- Examination
  - BMI, blood pressure, neck circumference
  - Body habitus, size of mandible/maxilla, retrognathia/prognathia, facial character
  - Nasal: size, deformity, valve, septum, turbinates, polyps/masses, adenoids
  - Oral Cavity/Oropharynx: size/position of tongue, elongated palate/uvula, tonsils, Mallampati score/Friedman classification, dentition, crowding of oral pharynx
  - Hypopharynx: size/position of tongue base, lingual tonsillar hypertrophy
  - Larynx: mobility of vocal cords, masses/polyps
  - Neck: size, placement of hyoid, jaw/retrognathia
  Flexible nasolaryngoscopy: awake, asleep, lying down
  - Müller maneuver: nose pinched close with mouth closed, inhale against closed airway examining retropalatal and retrolingual areas for collapse
- Drug-induced sleep videoendoscopy: a powerful tool for studying the dynamic airway in a sleeping patient.
  - Propofol-induced sleep
  - Evaluate degree of obstruction from lateral pharyngeal folds, retropalatal area, retrolingual area
- Imaging
  - Lateral radiographic cephalometry
  Inferiorly displaced hyoid, small posterior airway space, long palate
    Mandibular plane to hyoid distance <21 mm associated with higher success in patients with mild to moderate OSA undergoing uvulopalatopharyngoplasty (UPPP)
- MRI: to evaluate soft tissue
- Fluoroscopy: can improve UPPP selection/outcomes
    Time intensive, radiation exposure

- *Nocturnal Polysomnography (PSG)*: Gold Standard

– Level 1:

Electroencephalogram (EEG)
Electro-oculogram (EOG)
Submental electromyogram (EMG)
Electrocardiogram (ECG)
Nasal and oral airflow
Thoracoabdominal effort
Blood oxygen concentration/Oximetry (SaO_2)
Body position
Snoring

– Level 2:

Unattended study performed in the patient's home, limited by lack of technician to perform hookup
Same measures as Level 1

– Level 3:

Unattended, same limitations as Level 2
Heart rate
Airflow
Oximetry
May underestimate AHI because does not determine sleep versus wake

– Level 4:

Unattended

1–2 parameters, including oxygen saturation

– Apnea–Hypopnea Index

AHI <5—Normal, Snoring, or Upper Airway Resistance Syndrome (UARS)
AHI 5–15—Mild Sleep Apnea
AHI 15–30—Moderate Sleep Apnea
AHI >30—Severe Sleep Apnea

Therapy
Conservative

- Behavioral Modifications
  - Avoid alcohol, sedatives at bedtime
  - Weight loss or bariatric surgery (for morbidly obese patients)
  - Positional therapy: supine position, tongue falls posteriorly enhancing obstruction
- Positive Airway Pressure ventilation
  1. CPAP (Continuous positive airway pressure): <u>Gold Standard</u>
     - Pneumatic splint, prevents upper airway collapse, constant intraluminal pressure during inspiration and expiration
  2. BiPAP
     - Separately adjustable lower expiratory and higher inspiratory PAP
  3. APAP (Autoadjusting PAP)
     - Autotitrate PAP to select an effective level of CPAP to prevent upper airway collapse
     - Pressure changes in response to variations, snoring, impedence
- Oral Appliances
  Mild to moderate OSA
  - Mobilizes mandible and base of tongue anteriorly, maintains patency of posterior oropharyngeal airway
  - Complicated by tooth/jaw pain, increase in salivation overnight, dry mouth
- Medications: insufficient evidence.
- Nasal Strips
  - Can decrease snoring, mouth breathing, sleepiness
  - Can improve UPPP selection/outcomes

Surgical: Determined by the site of obstruction

- Nasal: can reduce CPAP requirements, rarely cures OSA [Septoplasty, Turbinate surgery, Nasal valve repair, Sinus surgery, Adenoidectomy]

- Palatal: UPPP with or without tonsillectomy
  - Transpalatal advancement pharyngoplasty after UPPP if persistent OSA: remove 1 cm of the hard palate, advance the soft palate, secure to tensor aponeurosis
  - Expansion sphincteroplasty: variation of UPPP
  - Uvulopalatal flap: reflecting the uvula and posterior portion of the soft palate anteriorly
  - Z-palatoplasty
  - Laser-assisted uvulopalatoplasty (LAUP): two vertical cuts in soft palate on either side of uvula, amputate lower two-thirds to three-fourths of the uvula. Scar retraction and stiffening of the palate is achieved
  - Cautery-assisted palatal stiffening (CAPSO): remove mucosa off midline of soft palate, induces scar tissue resulting in stiffer palate
  - Radiofrequency ablation of soft palate: soft palate coagulation necrosis causes scarring and contraction of tissue, shorter stiffer soft palate
  - Palate implant: 3–5 implantable rods inserted into the palate for scar formation
  - Injection snoreplasty: inject sclerosing agent (alcohol, sodium tetradecyl sulfate) into midline of soft palate
- Tongue Base
  - Partial midline glossectomy
    CO_2 laser, electrocautery, plasma knife, coblation
    Risk of bleeding from lingual artery, hypoglossal nerve injury, hematoma, abscess, dysphagia, taste disturbance
  - Lingualplasty
  - Lingual tonsillectomy
  - Radiofrequency tongue base ablation
    Four lesions at circumvallate papilla to reduce tissue volume at the tongue base
- Hypopharyngeal
  - Genioglossus advancement
    More anteriorly positioned tongue with increased tension on the genioglossus
      Rectangular geniotubercle osteotomy with advancement
      Risk of dental root injury, mandible fracture, hematoma

- Hyoid myotomy/suspension
  Hyoid mobilized anteriorly and superiorly via attachment to the mandible or to thyroid cartilage
    Risk of numbness, infection, seroma, fracture, death
- Tongue suspension
- Base of tongue to anterior floor of mouth
  - <u>Maxillomandibular advancement</u>
    Most effective surgical procedure for OSA
      Enlarges pharyngeal and hypopharyngeal airway
      Risk of malocclusion, relapse, nerve paresthesia, nonunion, malunion, temporomandibular joint tenderness, infection
- Tracheotomy
  - Bypass the site of upper airway obstruction
  - Indications: morbid obesity, arrhythmia with apnea, severe apnea with desaturation, cor pulmonale, no response to dietary modifications or CPAP, chronic alveolar hypoventilation

Further Readings

1. Johannesen KM, Bodtger U. Lemierre's syndrome: current perspectives on diagnosis and management. Infect Drug Resist. 2016;9:221–7.
2. Burton MJ, Pollard AJ, Ramsden JD, Chong LY, Venekamp RP. Tonsillectomy for periodicfever, aphthous stomatitis, pharyngitis and cervical adenitis syndrome (PFAPA). Cochrane Database Syst Rev. 2014;9:CD008669.

Chapter 10
Oral Cavity

10.1 Congenital Epulis (Granular Cell Tumor)

A benign intraoral tumour present in the mucosa of the alveolar ridge.

Symptoms

It can lead to difficulties during food ingestion.

Diagnosis

– Light-red neoplasm on the oral mucosa.
– X-ray: Shows erosion of the bony alveolar processes.

Therapy

– Surgical excision (including the periosteum).

10.2 Torus Palatinus and Mandibularis

Bony exostoses, located along the midline of the hard palate (torus palatinus) and on the lingual surface of the mandible (torus mandibularis).

P. Koltsidopoulos et al., *ENT*,
DOI 10.1007/978-3-319-56330-5_10,
© Springer International Publishing AG 2017

Treatment is only required when:

1. the lesion interferes with the fitting of the dentures
2. the exostosis has recurrent infections,
3. ulceration or
4. neoplasm.

10.3   Ankyloglossia

Short lingual frenulum, which fixes the tongue to the floor of mouth.

– Difficulties with breastfeeding related to poor weight gain, excessively long feeds.
– Difficulties with speech

Therapy

– Division of the frenulum.

10.4   Lingual Thyroid

In cases of failure of thyroid migration, the thyroid gland may persist in the lingual base.

Symptoms

– Dysphagia
– Lump-in-throat sensation
– Dyspnoea
– Speech affection.
– Patients could be hypothyroid.

Diagnosis

• Inspection: a mass in the base of the tongue. Diagnosis can occur during hypermetabolic conditions (pregnancy, infections, trauma, and menopause) because of the increased size of the gland.

- When lingual thyroid is suspected, normal thyroid tissue should be searched.
- Thyroid function tests, cervical ultrasound and thyroid scanning should be undertaken.

Therapy

- Suppression with thyroid hormone to decrease the size of the lingual thyroid.
- Radioactive iodine ablation
- Surgical excision (severe symptoms).

10.5 Fissured Tongue

A condition characterized by grooves and fissures of varying depth on the dorsal surface of the tongue.

- The incidence is 10–20%.
- Autosomal-dominant hereditary component is presumed. It can be combined with Melkersson–Rosenthal syndrome, Down's syndrome or acromegaly.
- Asymptomatic.
- The fissures may occur laterally, medially or are spread all over the tongue.
- No therapy is necessary.

10.6 Geographic Tongue

A benign recurrent condition of uncertain aetiology affecting the tongue. It is characterized by delineated areas of shiny, erythematous mucosa in different regions of the tongue, surrounded by white borders.

- The lesion persists for a period of time and disappears only to reappear at a different location giving a different pattern.
- No clinical symptoms, except burning of the tongue and gustatory relay or loss in some cases.
- The tongue has irregular-shaped white and red spots. The fields move along the tongue.
- No treatment if asymptomatic
- Application of vitamin A and zinc.

10.7   Black Hairy Tongue

Clinical condition characterized by elongated filiform lingual papillae, which look like hairs on the dorsum of the tongue.

- Predisposing conditions: smoking, excessive coffee or black tea drinking, poor oral hygiene, dry mouth, drugs (antibiotics), chronic mucosal irritation and metabolic imbalance.
- Patients usually do not complain of any symptom. Rarely associated with burning mouth syndrome, dysgeusia, xerostomia, and halitosis.
- Diagnosis: inspection → Black surface of the tongue having a hairy appearance.
- Treatment: mechanical debridement, maintenance of proper oral hygiene, and removal of potential causative agents.

10.8   Hunter's Glossitis

Atrophic glossitis related to pernicious anaemia.

- The tongue shows an atrophic inflammation.

Symptoms

Burning of the tongue, paraesthesia, and dry mouth.

Diagnosis

1. Inspection: The surface of the tongue is atrophic and glazed.
2. The serum level of vitamin B12 must be measured.

Therapy

In the case of a low concentration, folic acid needs to be substituted.

10.9   Syphillis

An infectious venereal disease caused by the spirochete Treponema pallidum.

- Routes of transmission: by sexual contact, from mother to fetus in utero, via blood product transfusion, and occasionally through breaks in the skin that come into contact with infectious lesions.
- Stages: Primary, secondary and tertiary syphilis may all occur in the oral cavity (especially primary and secondary).
  - **Primary**: a single painless chancre occurs after incubation period of 2–3 weeks. Extra-genitallocalizations are the lips, the tongue, buccal mucosa and the hard and the soft palate.
  - **Secondary**: a skin eruption of various appearances with mucous patches occurs on the lips and intraorally. There is latency of between 4 and 6 months. These lesions are often painful. The patches are highly communicable because of the high bacterial concentration.
  - **Tertiary**: Formation of a gumma starts after 3–10 years. Gummas are painless, well-defined ulcers. Healing with scar formation is possible.

Diagnosis

- Microbial detection is possible in primary syphilis by dark-field microscopy.
- Serologic tests for syphilis verify the diagnosis (Treponema pallidum haemagglutination test, fluorescent treponemal antibody absorption/FTA-Abs) are necessary in cases of secondary and tertiary syphilis.

<u>Differential Diagnosis</u>: neoplasm, specific angina-like mononucleosis, Vincent's angina and diphtheria.

Therapy

- Primary, secondary and latent syphilis (duration of infection less than 1 year): benzathine penicillin G or procaine penicillin intramuscularly.
- Alternative therapy with doxycycline or erythromycin in penicillin-allergic patients.
- In tertiary and latent syphilis (duration of infection more than 1 year) benzathine penicillin intramuscularly

10.10   Actinomycosis

Infection caused by Actinomycetes bacteria.

Symptoms

- Starts as a painless nodule, which is located in the mucosal and submucosal tissues. Often the nodule erupts intra-orally or to the surface of the skin. Patients present with swelling and erythematous skin or mucosa.

Complications

- Chronic draining fistula persists, especially when the submandibular or the parotid gland are infected.

Therapy

- Penicillin therapy for a long time: penicillin G iv for 4–6 weeks, after that penicillin V or amoxicillin for 6–12 months.

10.11   Submandibular Space Abscess (Ludwig's Angina)

An aggressive, rapidly spreading, bilateral, indurated cellulitis occurring in the suprahyoid soft tissues, the floor of the mouth, and both sublingual and submandibular spaces.

<u>Etiological factors</u>: infection of second or third mandibular molar tooth, extension of peritonsillar cellulitis, poor dental hygiene, tooth extractions, trauma, injury to oral mucosa, lingual tonsillitis or salivary gland disease.
- Infection can spread to the deeper neck spaces, to the submandibular, parapharyngeal and retropharyngeal spaces.

Symptoms

- High fever
- Pain in floor of mouth
- Trismus
- Drooling
- Patients cannot speak or swallow because of tongue involvement.
- Oedema, submandibular induration, tenderness and swelling are evident.

Complications

- Airway obstruction
- Infection to the mediastinum

Diagnosis

- Clinical examination: the skin beneath the chin is erythematous and oedematous; the oedema can be spread down onto the skin of the anterior neck and descend onto the chest wall.
- Complete blood counts.
- Bacterial cultures.
- CT scan/US: to assess the extension of an abscess

Therapy

Conservative treatment
- Airway control: maintenance of a safe and secure airway is mandatory
- Prompt antibiotic therapy

Surgical treatment:

1. If there is obvious abscess formation
2. If anaerobic bacteria are present, seen by gas within the soft tissues in the CT scans (indicating aggressive anaerobic fasciitis).
3. If there is no improvement after conservative treatment.

<u>Surgical procedures</u>

- Submandibular and submental space is opened through horizontal incision paralleling the mandible. All loculated areas of the abscess must be opened and drained.
- During surgery bacterial cultures and biopsies should be obtained.
- After surgery monitoring of the number of white blood cells and the fever is required. If they do not decrease, another occult abscess cavity exists and the CT scans should be repeated. In case of a residual abscess, a further surgical drainage is necessary.
- Tracheotomy or nasopharyngeal intubation may be necessary to control the airway.
- Removal of the infected teeth needs to be done.

10.12   Mucosal Candidiasis

Pathogen: **Candida albicans**

<u>Risk groups</u>: Patients with immune deficiencies (organ transplants, HIV, diabetes, radiation therapy and long-term antibiotic or corticoid therapy).

Symptoms

- Dysphagia
- Sore throat and painful swallowing

Diagnosis

- Physical examination: Red, irregular and flat lesions in oral cavity. Sometimes there are white plaques with a red margin, which start bleeding on scraping the plaques.
- Gram stain or culture: to confirm diagnosis

Therapy

- Topic antifungal medication: nystatin or clotrimazole
- In severe cases systemic application of fluconazole.

10.13   Herpetic Gingival Stomatitis

- Mainly caused by HSV-1. Infections of HSV-2 are usually located in genital regions.
- Route of transmission: usually direct contact or droplet transmission.
- The incidence in adults is 85–90%.
- The incubation period is 5–7 days.
- In most cases initial infection happens in childhood and has its manifestation in the oral cavity.
- The virus persists after initial infection in ganglionic cells after primary infection.

Symptoms

A. Primary manifestation
   - Gingival and oral mucosa are erythematous.
   - Characteristic low-grade fever, malaise and lymphadenitis.
   - Vesicular lesions occur in the oral cavity, erupt within 24 h and live flat, grey ulcers with a halo-sign appearance. Erosions heal after 1 week without scar formation.
   - Young patients present with fetor, hypersalivation and painful food ingestion.

B. Reactivated infection
   - Reactivation of the virus occurs as labial herpes (triggered by pregnancy, stress, sunlight or feverish infections).

- Favoured manifestation is at the mucocutaneous border of the lips, sometimes the nasal vestibule, the cheeks or the eyelids. Clinical symptoms are paraesthesia, burning skin and mucosa; within a few hours crops of vesicular lesions occur.

Complications

- "Pospischill–Feyrter disease" (vesicular lesions spread all over the facial skin): in patients with immunosuppression
- Bacterial superinfection with staphylococcior streptococci.
- Meningitis

Diagnosis

- Based on clinical symptoms.
- It can be established by assay, but it is very expensive.

Therapy

- The virus cannot be eliminated; early treatment with antiviral medication is necessary to decrease the viral load.
- Primary infection: 5×200 mg aciclovir per day orally for 10–14 days.
- Reactivated infection: topical application of penciclovir or aciclovir is necessary. Local aseptic treatment to avoid bacterial infection.

- Prognosis
  - Self-limited disease. Certain patients suffer from recurring infections.

10.14   Herpes Zoster

- The first contact with varicella zoster virus causes chickenpox (during childhood).
- Dormant VZV persists in ganglionic cells (trigeminal nerveganglion) in a latent state. It may be reactivated and affect the area of the nerve.

<u>Predisposing factors</u>: immunodeficiencies (HIV infection and immune-depressing therapy).

Symptoms

- Vesicular lesions similar to chickenpox arise in a dermatomal distribution on one side. The areas innervated by the second and third division of the trigeminal nerve are affected.
- <u>When the maxillary branch is affected</u>: lesions occur ipsi-laterally on the soft and the hard palate, on the uvula and on maxillary gingiva.
- <u>When the mandibular n. is affected</u>: lesions occur at the mucosa of the lower lip, the tongue and the floor of the mouth. Nearly all patients present with neuralgic pain before vesicular lesions can be seen.

Diagnosis

- Clinical symptoms verify the diagnosis.

Therapy

Therapy is useful if it is started within 3 days after lesions occur!
- Aciclovir orally 5 × 800 mg for 7–10 days (to decrease the intensity of the infection and the neuralgic pain).
- High-dose steroids
- Eye care
- Analgesics
- In case of postinfectious neuralgia, amitriptyline and car-bamazepine are helpful.

10.15   Herpangina

Infection with Coxsackie A virus.

- Children up to 7 years are mostly affected.

Symptoms

- Fever, headache and pharyngitis.

- Characteristic symptoms: Severe sore throat, excessive salivation and nausea.
  Small vesicles on the soft palate occur later on. They are surrounded by a red margin and erupt early. The vesicles are marked by crops of flat lesions on the tonsils, the soft palate and the uvula.

Diagnosis

- Clinical symptoms verify the diagnosis.

Differential Diagnosis

- Herpesvirus infection: affection of the whole gingiva during HSV infection, more severe symptomatology
- Aphthous stomatitis
- Bacterial pharyngitis
- Viral enanthema like chickenpox or measles.

Therapy

- Self-limited process
- Symptomatic therapy: oral treatment with local anaesthetics and silver nitrate (to accelerate the healing).

10.16   Hairy Leucoplakia

A benign, asymptomatic, white, hyperkeratotic lesion affecting primarily the lateral border of the tongue, unilaterally or bilaterally.

- It affects immunocompromised patients (HIV, post-transplantation patients).
- It is a pathognomonic sign for HIV; this condition heralds the onset of full-blown acquired immunodeficiency syndrome (AIDS).

Symptoms

- A shaggy appearance of the tongue is apparent and may vary in colour from white to grey to black.

- Preferred localization: the lateral margins of tongue. The lesion may spread to dorsum and ventral surfaces.

Therapy

- Symptomatic treatment

10.17   Kaposi's Sarcoma

- The most frequent HIV-associated oral malignancy
- Its incidence has dramatically decreased in the potent anti-retroviral therapy era
- In 90% of all HIV-associated Kaposi's sarcomas, HHV type 8 can be found.
- May occur long before other opportunistic infections.

Symptoms

A. Early phase: cutaneous and lymphatic affection
B. Advanced stage: gastrointestinal or/and pulmonal affection, sometimes with extensive oral affection.
   - Skin and especially oral mucosa show red to livid macules, plaques or nodes; sometimes they are confluent.

Diagnosis

- Inspection
- Palpation (lymph nodes!)
- Blood examination
- Biopsy: to verify the diagnosis.

Therapy

- It is very important to optimize the antiretroviral therapy.
- Sarcoma can be regressive or disappear completely.

Therapeutic options according to the stage of the disease

- Limited cutaneous sarcoma: Radiotherapy, laser therapy or cryotherapy, surgical removal.
- Disseminated sarcoma: Systemic therapy with α-interferon.

Success depends on the level of CD4 cells at the beginning.

10.18   Aphthous Stomatitis

- Disorder of unknown etiology.
- The disease may be familiar.
- The preferred age is between 20 and 30 years.
- Predisposing factors: stress and hormonal imbalance.

Symptoms

- Multiple spherical flat craterlike lesions form in the mobile mucosa of the oral cavity.

Three clinical variants:

1. <u>Minor type (Mikulicz)</u> (80–90%): superficial little (2–5 mm) aphthous ulcers in the anterior part of the oral cavity; healing occurs without scar formation within 1 week.
2. <u>Major type (Sutton)</u> (10%): The ulcers are more extended (1–4 cm) and infiltrate the mucosa. Preferred localizations are the tongue and the lips; a pseudomembrane covers the crater.

   The defect heals within 2 weeks with scar formation. Mostly, disease is accompanied by lymphadenitis.
3. <u>Herpetiform type</u> (5%): very small lesions, with less symptoms.

Differential Diagnosis

Behçet's syndrome and herpesvirus infection.

Therapy

- Local anaesthetics
- Local corticoid treatment (such as Volon A salve)
- Aseptic agents.

10.19   Pemphigus Vulgaris

It is a potentially fatal autoimmune, intraepithelial disease characterized by flaccid blisters and erosions of the skin and mucous membranes.

- It is a disease with antibodies targeted against the desmosomes of the epithelium leading to bullous desquamation and supraepithelial split with Tzanck cells.

Symptoms

- In half of the patients oral manifestation occurs.
- Oral cavity is spread with blisters, filled with bloody or serous discharge. Within hours the blisters erupt and flat lesions occur. Primarily the lesions are not painful, but after eruption the pain is severe.
- Odynophagia and throat and tongue pain.

Diagnosis

- Biopsy with immuno-fluorescent stain in order to detect the antibodies.
- Antibodies can be found in the skin and mucosal areas as well as in the serum.

Therapy

- Systemic corticosteroids in combination with immunosuppressants (azathioprine, methotrexate).
- The disease may be lethal if it stays unchecked and untreated.

10.20 Pemphigoid

Pemphigoid is an autoimmune subepidermal blistering dermatosis.

It features circulating autoantibodies against distinctive skin's basal membrane antigens and adjacent mucous membrane's antigens.

Symptoms

- Oral mucosa involvement most common in head and neck region, followed by ocular, nasal (25–50%, affects anterior nasal cavity), and nasopharyngeal.

Diagnosis

– Histology is used to verify the diagnosis (detection of colloid bodies in the lower epithelial layers).

Therapy

If multiple sites involved – dapsone for 12 weeks; can use topical corticosteroids for isolated oral mucosal involvement

10.21   Lichen Ruber Planus

A chronic and T-cell-mediated autoimmune disease with unknown aetiology.

The use of specific medication and stress seem to trigger the disease.

Multiple varieties of lichen planus exist. The most common form in the oral cavity is the reticular form.

Symptoms

Reticular form

– Occurs on the mucosa and on the skin at the same time. In 25–70% of cases the oral mucosa is associated with it.
– On the buccal mucosa, the lips and tongue, a lacelike reticular pattern of white lines appears (Wickham lines)

Erosive form

– Patients show no symptoms, except they present with an erosive form, which is very painful.

Diagnosis

– Histology is used to verify the diagnosis (detection of colloid bodies in the lower epithelial layers).

Differential Diagnosis

In the case of erosive lesions: Pemphigus vulgaris, syphilis and systemic lupus erythematosus.

Therapy

The disease is self-limited and requires the use of topical steroids to prevent scarring.
Retinoin and isoretinoin are useful in some cases.

10.22   Systemic Lupus Erythematous

A chronic systemic disease of the vasculature with involvement of the skin and the possibility of the affection of all other organs.

In 40% of cases the oral mucosa is involved.

Symptoms

- Intraorally discoid erythematous lesions occur, sometimes ulcerating.
- The butterfly rash of the facial skin over the nose and the cheeks is characteristic.
- General symptoms: Fever, muscular pain and involvement of the CNS and the kidney.

Diagnosis

- A complex blood and histologic examination is necessary;
- A dermatologist should be involved.
- Generally, antinuclear antibodies can be detected.

Therapy

- Topical and systemic application of steroids
- Therapy lies in the hand of the dermatologist.

10.23   Lymphomatoid Granulomatosis (Lethal Midline Granuloma)

- Considered to be a located muco-cutaneous T-cell lymphoma.

- Erosions of hard palate occur, generally in the area of the junction.

Symptoms

- Ulceration of mucosal surfaces, in both the nose and the sinus. In some cases, the oral cavity is also affected.

Therapy

- Low-dose radiation;
- In systemic cases chemotherapy.
- The disease has a high mortality rate (50–70% over a 5-year period).

10.24   Necrotizing Sialometaplasia

An uncommon benign reactive necrotizing inflammatory process involving mainly the minor salivary glands.

- It occurs as a necrotizing, painful ulcer with deep infiltration.
- It is found on the junction of the soft and the hard palate
- It often mimics carcinoma.
- The palate and the nose may be perforated and destructed.

Diagnosis

Biopsy: easy to mistake as malignancy histopathologically.

Therapy

- Topically applied lidocaine.
- Self-resolution.

10.25   Behcet's Syndrome

A systemic inflammatory disease involving primarily the oral and genital mucosa, skin and eyes.

- Unknown cause (auto-immune or viral origin is speculated).
- It occurs often in male patients in eastern countries such as Turkey.

Symptoms–Diagnosis
Diagnosis is based on the following diagnostic criteria:

Major symptoms:
Recurrent oral aphthous ulcers, recurrent genital ulcers, skin lesions and uveitis.

Minor symptoms:
Arthritis, gastrointestinal symptoms and vasculitis.

Therapy

- Immunosuppressants: cyclophosphamide, colchicines and steroids
- Topical steroids and analgesics

10.26   Melkersson-Rosenthal Syndrome

A rare neurological disorder characteristic by fissured tongue, granulomatous cheilitis and recurrent facial palsy

- Swelling of the upper lip, lower lip, or one or both cheeks is usually the first symptom
- The first episode may resolve in hours or days, but swelling may be more severe and last longer in subsequent episodes and can become permanent.

Diagnosis

- Physical findings and history
- Lip biopsy: to confirm the diagnosis in some cases

Therapy

- Steroids

10.27   Angioedema

Angioedema is defined by swelling of the skin or mucosal tissues, resulting from temporary increase in vascular permeability.

1. Hereditary (deficiency of C1 inhibitor)
2. Acquired (associated with other diseases)
3. Allergic
4. Drug-induced (ACE inhibitors or NSAIDs)
5. Idiopathic

Symptoms

- Swelling in tongue, lips, throat
- Airway blockage

Diagnosis

- Detailed history
- Cutaneous or in vitro testing for immediate hypersensitivity
- Measurement of C4 level, C1 INH antigenic level and C1 INH functional level.

Therapy

- Epinephrine (may be life-saving when angioedema is allergic).
- Antihistamines
- Leucotriene receptor antagonists (montelukast)
- Corticosteroids
- Agents used in treating HAE:
  C1 INH concentrates, ecallantide, and icatibant

Surgical therapy

- In severe cases of laryngeal edema, tracheotomy may be required.

10.28 Burning Mouth Syndrome

Burning sensation in the oral mucosa without findings on physical examination.

Etiology

<u>Primary</u>: unknown etiology

<u>Secondary</u>:

- Endocrine disorders (menopause, thyroid hypofunction)
- Allergies to dental products, dental materials or foods
- Dry mouth, which can be caused by certain disorders (such as Sjögren's syndrome) and treatments (such as certain drugs and RT)
- Iatrogenic (angiotensin-converting enzyme (ACE) inhibitors and angiotensin receptor blockers (ARBs)
- Nutritional deficiencies (such as a low level of vitamin B, iron, zinc, and folate)
- Infection in the mouth
- Acid reflux

Symptoms

- Pain in the mouth that is burning,
- scalding, or tingling.
- dry mouth or altered taste.

Diagnosis

Diagnosis of BMS is based on following steps:

- To rule-out history of pain
- To check through clinical examination
- Information on previous or current psychosocial and psychological well-being
- To measure salivary flow rates and taste function
- Neurological imaging and examine the pathology and degenerative disorders
- Oral cultures to confirm suspected infections
- Patch test for allergic individuals

- Gastric reflux studies
- Hematological test to rule out nutritional, hormonal, auto-immune conditions.

Therapy

- Antidepressants, analgesics, antiepileptic, antifungal, antibacterial, sialagogues, antihistamines, anxiolytics, antipsychotics and vitamin, mineral, and hormonal replacements.

Further Readings

1. McMillan R, Taylor J, Shephard M, Ahmed R, Carrozzo M, Setterfield J, Grando S, Mignogna M, Kuten-Shorrer M, Musbah T, Elia A, McGowan R, Kerr AR, Greenberg MS, Hodgson T, Sirois D. World Workshop on Oral Medicine VI: a systematic review of the treatment of mucocutaneous pemphigus vulgaris. Oral Surg Oral Med Oral Pathol Oral Radiol. 2015;120(2): 132–42.
2. Imbery TA, Edwards PA. Necrotizing sialometaplasia: literature review and case reports. J Am Dent Assoc. 1996;127(7):1087–92.
3. Hatemi G, Seyahi E, Fresko I, Talarico R, Hamuryudan V. One year in review 2016: Behçet's syndrome. Clin Exp Rheumatol. 2016;34(6 Suppl 102):10–22.
4. Bas M. The angiotensin-converting-enzyme-induced angio-edema. Immunol Allergy Clin N Am. 2017;37(1):183–200.
5. McMillan R, Forssell H, Buchanan JA, Glenny AM, Weldon JC, Zakrzewska JM. Interventions for treating burning mouth syndrome. Cochrane Database Syst Rev. 2016;18:11.

Chapter 11
Thyroid and Parathyroid Glands

Ten Thyroid Anatomy Pearls

1. <u>Pyramidal lobe</u>: a remnant of descent of the thyroid that usually arises from the isthmus. Present in up to 40% of population.
2. <u>Posterior suspensory ligament of the thyroid (ligament of Berry)</u>: a condensation of the thyroid fascia. It is well vascularized, deriving a branch of the inferior thyroid artery.
3. <u>Internal branch of superior laryngeal nerve (SLN)</u>: supplies sensation to the lower pharynx, supraglottic larynx, and base of tongue.
4. The internal branch of SLN travels medially to the carotid system, entering the posterior aspect of the thyrohyoid membrane.
5. <u>External branch of SLN</u>: provides motor innervation to the cricothyroid muscle.
6. The SLN's external branch diverges from the superior pole vascular pedicle 1 cm or more above the superior aspect of the thyroid superior pole.
7. <u>Recurrent laryngeal nerve (RLN)</u>: provides motor innervation to the inferior constrictor and all intrinsic laryngeal muscles except the cricothyroid.

P. Koltsidopoulos et al., *ENT*,
DOI 10.1007/978-3-319-56330-5_11,
© Springer International Publishing AG 2017

8. The right RLN ascends the neck, traveling from lateral to medial, crossing the inferior thyroid artery.
9. The left RLN ascends in a more paratracheal position, crossing the distal branches of the inferior thyroid artery.
10. <u>Tubercle of Zuckerkandl</u>: a pyramidal extension of the thyroid gland, present at the most posterior side of each lobe. It is a reliable landmark for the RLN in thyroid surgery.

Non-malignantthyroid Disorders

11.1   Graves Disease

Autoimmune thyroid disease characterized by production of immunoglobulins that bind and activate TSH receptors, leading to continuous and uncontrolled thyroid stimulation → ↑TH.

– Women aged 40–60 years have the highest risk of developing the disease.

Symptoms

– Diffuse enlargement of thyroid (goiter).
– Symptoms of hyperthyroidism (weight loss, heat sensitivity, moist skin, anxiety and irritability, erectile dysfunction, tremor, frequent bowel movements)
– Infiltrative opthalmopathy (exophthalmos).
– Infiltrative dermopathy (localized myxedema, thick, red skin)
– Osteopathy

Diagnosis

- Blood tests: lower than normal levels of TSH and higher levels of thyroid hormones
- Radioactive iodine uptake: diffuse increased gland uptake.

Therapy

- Radioactive iodine ablation
- Antithyroid drugs
- Beta blockers (block the effect of hormones on the body)
- Surgery

11.2 Subacute Thyroiditis (deQuervain's)

> Acute inflammatory disease of the thyroid probably caused by a virus.

- The most common cause of painful thyroid.
- Viral in etiology.

Symptoms

- Enlarged and painful thyroid, often after URI.
- Fever and malaise are common.

Diagnosis

- Primary clinical
- Transient hyperthyroidism.
- 50% will enter a hypothyroid phase lasting several months.

Therapy

- Self-limiting disease.
- NSAIDs and rarely steroids.

11.3   Hashimoto Thyroiditis

A thyroid autoimmune disease causing hypothyroidism.

Symptoms

- Painless, firm, symmetric goiter
- Symptoms of hypothyroidism

Complications

- Thyroid lymphoma (rare)

Diagnosis

- Elevated levels of thyroid peroxidase antibodies (70–90%) anti-TPO
- Usually euthyroid at presentation. Hypothyroidism may develop with time.

Therapy

- Hypothyroid patients: thyroxine replacement therapy.
- Large, symptomatic goiter causing pressure symptoms or refractive to TH: surgery

11.4   Multinodular Goiter

The commonest thyroid gland disorder.

Symptoms

- Mass in the neck
- Pressure symptoms: Dysphagia, Choking sensation, Inspiratory stridor

Therapy

- Long term suppressive therapy
- Treatment with 131I or surgery.

11.5   Thyroid Cancer

Papillary (80%): Often multicentric both within ipsilateral and contralateral lobe.

- The 20-year survival rate is very high.
- It spreads to central and lateral lymph nodes.
- Cervical metastatic disease does not usually affect prognosis
- Pathological findings: "Orphan Annie eye" nucleus
- Total thyroidectomy
- Lobectomy is acceptable for microcarcinomas (<1.0 cm)
- Central compartment ND: regional metastases or in high-risk patients

Follicular (10–15%):

- The 20-year survival rate is approximately 70%.
- May exhibit minimal or wide vascular invasion, which affects prognosis
- Primarily hematogenous or direct spread with little lymphatic invasion
- It can metastasize via hematologic pathways and spread to the lungs, liver, bones.
- Total thyroidectomy followed by 131I ablation

Huerthle cell (2%): aggressive variant of follicular carcinoma.

- 20% present with cervical lymph node metastases, 10% present with distant metastases (bones, lung).
- Total thyroidectomy
- Central ND in the presence of regional metastases.

Medullary (5–10%): It originates from the C cells of the thyroid that secrete calcitonin.

- 75% occur sporadically and 25% are familial in origin.
- It is often component of Multiple Endocrine Neoplasia syndromes types 2A and 2B (mutation of RET proto-oncogene).

- Genetic component → RET testing recommended
- Total thyroidectomy with central ND + selective ND.

Anaplastic (1%): Highly lethal cancer

- It usually arises from a well-differentiated thyroid carcinoma.
- It often metastasizes regionally as well as distally (lungs, liver, bones).
- Palliative therapy with RT and CT.
- Tracheotomy and gastrostomy tube placement are often required.

11.6   Management of Thyroid Nodules

- History.
  - Age ‹20 and ›60 years
  - Male gender
  - Rapid growth, pain
  - History of radiation exposure
  - Family history of thyroid carcinoma
  - Hard, fixed lesion
  - Vocal cord paralysis
  - Cervical nodules,
  - Size ›4 cm
  - Aerodigestive tract compromise
- Measurement of serum TSH
- Serum calcitonin levels if concerned about medullary thyroid cancer
- Ultrasound: allows identification, characterization, and trending of nodules, central and lateral lymphadenopathy
  - Findings suggesting malignancy: solid/hypoechoic appearance, increased vascularity, microcalcifications, irregular margins, absence of "halo" sign
- Ultrasound-guided FNA: improves diagnostic yield and selection of appropriate nodules to aspirate
  - Typically recommended for nodules >1 cm unless high-risk factors

Bethesda System

1. Non-diagnostic
2. Benign
3. Atypia of undetermined significance
4. Follicular neoplasm or suspicious for a suspicious neoplasm.
5. Suspicious for malignancy
6. Malignant

> **Three Parathyroid Anatomy Pearls**
>
> 1. Inferior glands arise from third pouch and migrate with thymus (Long descent → large area of possible ectopic placement).
>   Superior glands arise from fourth pouch (Shorter descent → much less variability).
> 2. Inferior: large area from angle of mandible to pericardium. Most common ectopic location anterior mediastinum
> 3. Superior: little variation in descent. Eighty-five percent can be found at posterior aspect of thyroid lobe in 1 cm above crossing of inferior thyroid artery and recurrent nerve

11.7   Primary Hyperparathyroidism (HPT)

> HPT is characterized by production and secretion of parathyroid hormone (PTH).

Causes

1. Single parathyroid adenoma
2. Double adenomas

3. Multigland hyperplasia
4. Carcinoma of parathyroid gland

Symptoms

- In many cases asymptomatic or vague symptoms
  Neurologic: Depression or mental confusion, sleep changes
  Renal: Kidney stones, hypercalciuria, polyuria-polydipsia
  Bone: bone and joint pain, osteopenia, osteoporosis, fractures, muscle weakness
  General symptoms: Abdominal pain, general aches and pains from no obvious cause, weight loss

Diagnosis

- Serum calcium levels: higher than normal
- PTH levels: to confirm the diagnosis of primary hyperparathyroidism
- Vitamin D, phosphorus, creatinine clearance, 24-h urine calcium
- Bone densitometry
- Neck imaging not indicated for diagnosis, but helpful for localization

Preoperative localization studies

- Parathyroid scintigraphy: Technetium 99 Sestamibi scanning
- High-resolution ultrasound: inexpensive and allows concurrent study of the thyroid gland
- MRI (Newer MRI has improved localization of adenomas especially for ectopic locations).
- Combination of techniques helps to increase sensitivity.

Therapy
Surgery

- Key to successful parathyroid adenoma is accurate preoperative localization
- Intraoperative parathyroid hormone (PTH) assay used at most centers to verify adequate treatment

<u>Complications</u>

- Persistent hyperparathyroidism
- Recurrent laryngeal nerve injury
- Transient postoperative hypocalcemia

11.8   Secondary Hyperparathyroidism

> Any disorder that results in hypocalcaemia will elevate parathyroid hormone levels and can serve as a cause of secondary HPT.

Etiology: the most frequent causes of the condition are chronic renal failure. Treatment is focused on treating the underlying disease.

11.9   Tertiary Hyperparathyroidism

> It occurs most commonly in the setting of renal transplant where patients with secondary HPT continue to have elevated PTH levels after receiving a renal allograft.

- This disease is observed in up to 30% of kidney transplant recipients.

Further Readings

1. Sheahan P, Murphy MS. Thyroid Tubercle of Zuckerkandl: importance in thyroid surgery. Laryngoscope. 2011;121(11):2335–7.
2. Tuluc M, Solomides C. Thyroid cytology. Otolaryngol Clin N Am. 2014;47(4):475–89.
3. Phitayakorn R, McHenry CR. Follicular and Hürthle cellcarcinoma of the thyroid gland. Surg Oncol Clin N Am. 2006;15(3):603–23, ix–x.

4. Kloos RT, et al. Medullary thyroid cancer: management guidelines of the American Thyroid Association. Thyroid. 2009;19(6):565–612.
5. Gioviale MC, Bellavia M, Damiano G, Lo Monte AI. Post-transplantation tertiaryhyperparathyroidism. Ann Transplant. 2012;17(3):111–9.

Chapter 12
Appendix

12.1 Tumor Staging - Oral Cavity, Oropharynx, Hypopharynx, Larynx, Paranasal Sinuses and Salivary Glands

Oral cavity	
TX	Primary tumor cannot be assessed
T0	No evidence of primary tumor
Tis	Carcinoma in situ
T1	Tumor 2 cm or less in greatest dimension
T2	Tumor more than 2 cm but not greater than 4 cm in greatest dimension
T3	Tumor more than 4 cm in greatest dimension
T4a	Moderately advanced local disease[a] Tumor invades through cortical bone, inferior alveolar nerve, floor of mouth, or skin of face—that is, chin or nose (oral cavity). Tumor invades adjacent structures (e.g., through cortical bone, into deep [extrinsic] muscle of tongue [genioglossus, hypoglossus, palataglos-sus, and styloglossus], maxillary sinus, skin of face)
T4b	Very advanced local disease Tumor invades masticator space, pterygoid plates, or skull base and/or encases internal carotid artery

[a]Note: Superficial erosion alone of bone/tooth socket by gingival primary is not sufficient to classify as T4

P. Koltsidopoulos et al., *ENT*,
DOI 10.1007/978-3-319-56330-5_12,
© Springer International Publishing AG 2017

Oropharynx

TX	Primary tumor cannot be assessed
T0	No evidence of primary tumor
Tis	Carcinoma in situ
T1	Tumor 2 cm or less in greatest dimension
T2	Tumor more than 2 cm but not greater than 4 cm in greatest dimension
T3	Tumor more than 4 cm in greatest dimension or extension to lingual surface of epiglottis
T4a	Moderately advanced local disease Tumor invades the larynx, deep/extrinsic muscle of the tongue, medial pterygoid, hard palate, or mandible[a]
T4b	Very advanced local disease Tumor invades the lateral pterygoid muscle, pterygoid plates, lateral nasopharynx, or skull base, or encases the carotid artery

[a]Note: Mucosal extension to lingual surface of epiglottis from primary tumors of the base of the tongue and vallecula does not constitute invasion of larynx

LARYNX—supraglottis

TX	Primary tumor cannot be assessed
T0	No evidence of primary tumor
Tis	Carcinoma in situ
T1	Tumor limited to one subsite of the supraglottis with normal vocal fold mobility
T2	Tumor invades mucosa of more than one adjacent subsite of the supraglottis or glottis or region outside the supraglottis (e.g., mucosa of base of tongue, vallecula, medial wall of pyriform sinus) without fixation of the larynx
T3	Tumor limited to the larynx with vocal fold fixation and/or invades any of the following: postcricoid area, pre-epiglottic tissues, paraglottic space, and/or inner cortex of thyroid cartilage

T4a	Moderately advanced local disease Tumor invades through the thyroid cartilage and/or invades tissues beyond the larynx (e.g., trachea, soft tissues of neck including deep extrinsic muscle of the tongue, strap muscles, thyroid, or esophagus)
T4b	Very advanced local disease Tumor invades prevertebral space, encases carotid artery, or invades mediastinal structures

LARYNX—glottis

TX	Primary tumor cannot be assessed
T0	No evidence of primary tumor
Tis	Carcinoma in situ
T1	Tumor limited to the vocal fold(s) (may involve anterior or posterior commissure) with normal mobility
T1a	Tumor limited to one vocal fold
T1b	Tumor involves both vocal folds
T2	Tumor extends to the supraglottis and/or subglottis, and/or with impaired vocal fold mobility
T3	Tumor limited to the larynx with vocal fold fixation and/or invasion of paraglottic space, and/or inner cortex of the thyroid cartilage
T4a	Moderately advanced local disease Tumor invades the outer cortex of the thyroid cartilage and/or invades tissues beyond the larynx (e.g., trachea, soft tissues of the neck, including deep extrinsic muscle of the tongue, strap muscles, thyroid, or esophagus)
T4b	Very advanced local disease Tumor invades prevertebral space, encases carotid artery, or invades mediastinal structures Subglottis

LARYNX—subglottis

TX	Primary tumor cannot be assessed
T0	No evidence of primary tumor
Tis	Carcinoma in situ
T1	Tumor limited to the subglottis
T2	Tumor extends to the vocal cord(s) with normal or impaired mobility
T3	Tumor limited to the larynx with vocal fold fixation
T4a	Moderately advanced local disease Tumor invades cricoid or thyroid cartilage and/or invades tissues beyond the larynx (e.g., trachea, soft tissues of the neck including deep extrinsic muscles of the tongue, strap muscles, thyroid, or esophagus)
T4b	Very advanced local disease Tumor invades prevertebral space, encases carotid artery, or invades mediastinal structures

Hypopharynx

TX	Primary tumor cannot be assessed
T0	No evidence of primary tumor
Tis	Carcinoma in situ
T1	Tumor limited to one subsite of the hypopharynx and is 2 cm or less in greatest dimension
T2	Tumor invades more than one subsite of the hypopharynx or an adjacent site, or measures more than 2 cm but not more than 4 cm in greatest dimension without fixation of the hemilarynx or extension to the esophagus
T3	Tumor more than 4 cm in greatest dimension or with fixation of the hemilarynx or extension to the esophagus
T4a	Moderately advanced local disease Tumor invades thyroid/cricoid cartilage, hyoid bone, thyroid gland, esophagus, or central compartment soft tissue[a]

| T4b | Very advanced local disease
Tumor invades prevertebral fascia, encases carotid artery, or involves mediastinal structures |

[a]Note: Central compartment soft tissue includes prelaryngeal strap muscles and subcutaneous fat

Maxillary sinus

TX	Primary tumor cannot be assessed
T0	No evidence of primary tumor
Tis	Carcinoma in situ
T1	Tumor limited to the maxillary sinus mucosa with no erosion or destruction of bone
T2	Tumor causing bone erosion or destruction, including extension into the hard palate and/or middle nasal meatus, except extension to the posterior wall of the maxillary sinus and pterygoid plates
T3	Tumor invades any of the following: bone of the posterior wall of the maxillary sinus, subcutaneous tissues, floor or medial wall of the orbit, pterygoid fossa, or ethmoid sinuses
T4a	Moderately advanced local disease Tumor invades anterior orbital contents, skin of cheek, pterygoid plates, infratemporal fossa, cribriform plate, sphenoid or frontal sinuses
T4b	Moderately advanced local disease Tumor invades any of the following: orbital apex, dura, brain, middle cranial fossa, cranial nerves other than maxillary division of trigeminal nerve (V), nasopharynx, or clivus

Ethmoid sinuses

TX	Primary tumor cannot be assessed
T0	No evidence of primary tumor
Tis	Carcinoma in situ

(continued)

(continued)

T1	Tumor restricted to any one subsite, with or without bony invasion
T2	Tumor invades two subsites in a single region or extending to involve an adjacent region within the nasoethmoidal complex, with or without bony invasion
T3	Tumor extends to invade the medial wall or floor of the orbit, maxillary sinus, palate, or cribriform plate
T4a	Moderately advanced local disease Tumor invades any of the following: anterior orbital contents, skin of nose or cheek, minimal extension to anterior cranial fossa, pterygoid plates, sphenoid or frontal sinuses
T4b	Very advanced local disease Tumor invades any of the following: orbital apex, dura, brain, middle cranial fossa, cranial nerves other than V, nasopharynx, or clivus

Salivary glands

TX	Primary tumor cannot be assessed
T0	No evidence of primary tumor
T1	Tumor 2 cm or less in greatest dimension without extraparenchymal extension
T2	Tumor greater than 2 cm but not more than 4 cm in greatest dimension without extraparenchymal extension[a]
T3	Tumor more than 4 cm and/or tumor having extraparenchymal extension
T4a	Moderately advanced local disease Tumor invades the skin, mandible, ear canal, and/or facial nerve
T4b	Very advanced local disease Tumor invades the skull base and/or pterygoid plates and/or encases the carotid artery

[a]Note: Extraparenchymal extension is a clinical macroscopic evidence of invasion of soft tissues. Microscopic evidence alone does not constitute extraparenchymal extension for classification purposes

Regional lymph nodes (N)

NX	Regional lymph nodes cannot be assessed
N0	No regional nodes metastasis
N1	Metastasis in a single ipsilateral lymph node, 3 cm or less in greatest dimension
N2a	Metastasis in a single ipsilateral lymph node, >3 cm and <6 cm
N2b	Metastasis in multiple ipsilateral lymph nodes, <6 cm
N2c	Metastasis in bilateral or contralateral lymph nodes, <6 cm
N3*	Metastasis in a lymph node more than 6 cm in greatest dimension

*A designation of "U" or "L" may be used for any N stage to indicate metastasis above the lower border of the cricoid cartilage (U) or below the lower border of the cricoid cartilage (L)

Distant metastasis (M)

MX	Distant metastasis cannot be assessed
M0	No distant metastasis
M1	Distant metastasis

TNM Staging for the Larynx, Oropharynx, Hypopharynx, Oral Cavity, Salivary Glands, and Paranasal Sinuses

Stage 0	Tis	N0	M0
Stage I	T1	N0	M0
Stage II	T2	N0	M0
Stage III	T3	N0	M0
	T1	N1	M0
	T2	N1	M0
	T3	N1	M0

(continued)

(continued)

Stage IVA	T4a	N0	M0
	T4a	N1	M0
	T1	N2	M0
	T2	N2	M0
	T3	N2	M0
	T4a	N2	M0
Stage IVB	Any T	N3	M0
	T4b	Any N	M0
Stage IVC	Any T	Any N	M1

12.2   Tumor Staging - Nasopharynx

Nasopharynx

TX	Primary tumor cannot be assessed
T0	No evidence of primary tumor
Tis	Carcinoma in situ
T1	Tumor confined to the nasopharynx or tumor extends to the oropharynx and/or nasal cavity without parapharyngeal extension
T2	Tumor with parapharygeal extension
T3	Tumor involves bony structures of skull base and/or paranasal sinuses
T4	Tumor with intracranial extension and/or involvement of cranial nerves, hypopharynx, orbit, or with extension to the infratemporal fossa/masticator space

Regional lymph nodes (N)

NX	Regional lymph nodes cannot be assessed
N0	No regional nodes metastasis

N1   Unilateral metastasis in cervical lymph node(s), 6 cm or less in greatest dimension, above the supraclavicular fossa, and/or unilateral or bilateral retropharyngeal lymph nodes, 6 cm or less in greatest dimension

N2   Bilateral metastasis in cervical lymph node(s), 6 cm or less in greatest dimension, above the supraclavicular fossa

N3   Metastasis in lymph node >6 cm and/or to supraclavicular fossa

N3a   Greater than 6 cm in dimension

N3b   Extension to the supraclavicular fossa

TNM Staging for Nasopharynx

Stage 0	Tis	N0	M0
Stage I	T1	N0	M0
Stage II	T2	N1	M0
	T2	N0	M0
	T2	N1	M0
Stage III	T1	N2	M0
	T2	N2	M0
	T3	N0	M0
	T3	N1	M0
	T3	N2	M0
Stage IVA	T4	N0	M0
	T4	N1	M0
	T4	N2	M0
Stage IVB	Any T	N3	M0
Stage IVC	Any T	Any N	M1

12.3   Tumor Staging - Thyroid Gland

Thyroid gland

TX	Primary tumor cannot be assessed
T0	No evidence of primary tumor
Tis	Carcinoma in situ
T1	Tumor 2 cm or less in greatest dimension, limited to the thyroid
T1a	Tumor 1 cm or less, limited to the thyroid
T1b	Tumor more than 1 cm but not more than 2 cm in greatest dimension, limited to the thyroid
T2	Tumor more than 2 cm but not more than 4 cm in greatest dimension, limited to the thyroid
T3	Tumor more than 4 cm in greatest dimension, limited to the thyroid or any tumor with minimal extrathyroid extension (e.g., extension to sternothyroid muscle or perithyroid soft tissues)
T4a	Moderately advanced local disease Tumor of any size extending beyond the thyroid capsule to invade subcutaneous soft tissues, larynx, trachea, esophagus, or recurrent laryngeal nerve
T4b	Very advanced local disease Tumor invades prevertebral fascia or encases the carotid artery or mediastinal vessels
T4a	Intrathyroidal anaplastic carcinoma (all anaplastic carcinomas are considered T4 tumors)
T4b	Extrathyroidal anaplastic* carcinoma with gross extrathyroid extension

*All anaplastic carcinomas are considered T4 tumors

REGIONAL LYMPH NODES (N)

NX	Regional lymph nodes cannot be assessed
N0	No regional nodes metastasis
N1	Regional lymph node metastasis

N1a	Metastasis to Level VI (pretracheal, paratracheal, and prelaryngeal/delphian lymph nodes)
N1b	Metastasis to unilateral, bilateral, or contralateral cervical Levels I, II, III, IV, or V) or superior mediastinal lymph nodes (Level VII)

Distant metastasis (M)

M0	No distant metastasis
M1	Distant metastasis

TNM staging for thyroid

Papillary or follicular carcinoma (differentiated)

Under 45 years

Stage I	Any T	Any N	M0
Stage II	Any T	Any N	M1

45 years and older

Stage I	T1	N0	M0
Stage II	T2	N0	M0
	T3	N0	M0
Stage III	T1	N1a	M0
	T2	N1a	M0
	T3	N1a	M0
Stage IVA	T4a	N0	M0
	T4a	N1a	M0
	T1	N1b	M0
	T2	N1b	M0
	T3	N1b	M0
	T4a	N1b	M0

(continued)

(continued)

Stage IVB	T4b	Any N	M0
Stage IVC	Any T	Any N	M1

Medullary carcinoma (all age groups)

Stage I	T1	N0	M0
Stage II	T2	N0	M0
	T3	N0	M0
Stage III	T1	N1a	M0
	T2	N1a	M0
	T3	N1a	M0
Stage IVA	T4a	N0	M0
	T4a	N1a	M0
	T1	N1b	M0
	T2	N1b	M0
	T3	N1b	M0
	T4a	N1b	M0
Stage IVB	T4b	Any N	M0
Stage IVC	Any T	Any N	M1

Anaplastic carcinoma

Stage IVA	T4a	Any N	M0
Stage IVB	T4b	Any N	M0
Stage IVC	Any T	Any N	M1

Index

P. Koltsidopoulos et al., *ENT*,
DOI 10.1007/978-3-319-56330-5,
© Springer International Publishing AG 2017

MIX
Papier aus verantwortungsvollen Quellen
Paper from responsible sources
FSC® C105338
FSC
www.fsc.org

If you have any concerns about our products,
you can contact us on
ProductSafety@springernature.com

In case Publisher is established outside the EU,
the EU authorized representative is:
Springer Nature Customer Service Center GmbH
Europaplatz 3, 69115 Heidelberg, Germany

Printed by Libri Plureos GmbH
in Hamburg, Germany